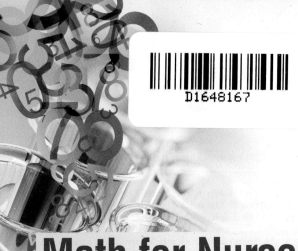

D1648167

Math for Nurses
A POCKET GUIDE TO DOSAGE CALCULATION AND DRUG PREPARATION

Mary Jo Boyer, RN, PhD

Vice Provost and Vice President
Branch Campus Operations
Adjunct Nursing Faculty
Former Dean and Professor of Nursing
Delaware County Community College
Media, Pennsylvania

Wolters Kluwer | Lippincott Williams & Wilkins
Health

Philadelphia • Baltimore • New York • London
Buenos Aires • Hong Kong • Sydney • Tokyo

Acquisitions Editor: Hilarie Surrena
Product Manager: Laura Scott
Design Coordinator: Joan Wendt
Illustration Coordinator: Brett MacNaughton
Manufacturing Coordinator: Karin Duffield
Prepress Vendor: Aptara, Inc.

8th edition

Copyright © 2013 Wolters Kluwer Health | Lippincott Williams & Wilkins.

Copyright © 2009 Wolters Kluwer Health | Lippincott Williams & Wilkins. Copyright © 2006 and 2002 Lippincott Williams & Wilkins. Copyright © 1998 Lippincott-Raven Publishers. Copyright © 1994 J.B. Lippincott Company. All rights reserved. This book is protected by copyright. No part of this book may be reproduced or transmitted in any form or by any means, including as photocopies or scanned-in or other electronic copies, or utilized by any information storage and retrieval system without written permission from the copyright owner, except for brief quotations embodied in critical articles and reviews. Materials appearing in this book prepared by individuals as part of their official duties as U.S. government employees are not covered by the above-mentioned copyright. To request permission, please contact Lippincott Williams & Wilkins at 2001 Market Street, Philadelphia, PA 19103, via email at permissions@lww.com, or via our website at lww.com (products and services).

9 8 7 6 5 4 3 2 1

Printed in China

Library of Congress Cataloging-in-Publication Data

Boyer, Mary Jo.
    Math for nurses : a pocket guide to dosage calculation and drug preparation / Mary Jo Boyer.—8th ed.
       p. ; cm.
    Includes bibliographical references and index.
    ISBN 978-1-60913-680-2 (alk. paper)
    I. Title.
    [DNLM: 1. Pharmaceutical Preparations–administration & dosage–Handbooks. 2. Pharmaceutical Preparations–administration & dosage–Nurses' Instruction. 3. Dosage Forms–Handbooks. 4. Dosage Forms–Nurses' Instruction. 5. Drug Dosage Calculations–Handbooks. 6. Drug Dosage Calculations–Nurses' Instruction. 7. Mathematics–Handbooks. 8. Mathematics–Nurses' Instruction. QV 735]
    LC classification not assigned
    615.1′4—dc23
                                              2011030507

CCS1211

Care has been taken to confirm the accuracy of the information presented and to describe generally accepted practices. However, the author, editors, and publisher are not responsible for errors or omissions or for any consequences from application of the information in this book and make no warranty, expressed or implied, with respect to the currency, completeness, or accuracy of the contents of the publication. Application of this information in a particular situation remains the professional responsibility of the practitioner; the clinical treatments described and recommended may not be considered absolute and universal recommendations.

The author, editors, and publisher have exerted every effort to ensure that drug selection and dosage set forth in this text are in accordance with the current recommendations and practice at the time of publication. However, in view of ongoing research, changes in government regulations, and the constant flow of information relating to drug therapy and drug reactions, the reader is urged to check the package insert for each drug for any change in indications and dosage and for added warnings and precautions. This is particularly important when the recommended agent is a new or infrequently employed drug.

Some drugs and medical devices presented in this publication have Food and Drug Administration (FDA) clearance for limited use in restricted research settings. It is the responsibility of the health care provider to ascertain the FDA status of each drug or device planned for use in his or her clinical practice.

LWW.com

Dedication

Math for Nurses was first published in 1987. At that time I was a professor of nursing at Delaware County Community College. Brian was 7 years old, and Susan was 12 months old. This is now the eighth edition. I've dedicated previous books to my students, professional colleagues, friends, and family. However, over the years, it is my family who has continued to energize, support, and encourage my academic and creative interests. So, for this edition, I salute, honor, and thank my family again for always being there.

Ermelina: my mother, who is 90 going on 75

Susan: a University of Richmond graduate, working in the finance world for the government in Washington, D.C.

Brian: a mathematics high school instructor, pursuing two master's degrees while also teaching at the college level

Kristen: my new daughter-in-law, who embraces family and faith as life's priorities

Sadie: my darling granddaughter, whose laughter lights up all of our lives

Bill: my husband and partner since 1974

Thanks Guys!

Contributors

Brian D. Boyer, AS, BA
Mathematics Instructor
Phoenixville High School
Phoenixville, Pennsylvania

Elaine Dreisbaugh, RN, MSN, CPN
Associate Professor of Nursing
Delaware County Community College
Media, Pennsylvania
Former Nurse Educator, The Chester County Hospital
West Chester, Pennsylvania

Kathleen C. Jones, RN, MSN, CDE
Certified Diabetic Nurse Educator
The Outpatient Diabetes Program
The Chester County Hospital
West Chester, Pennsylvania

Joanne O'Brian, RN, MSN
Associate Professor of Nursing
Delaware County Community College
Media, Pennsylvania
Nurse Educator, The Chester County Hospital
West Chester, Pennsylvania

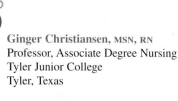

Reviewers

Ginger Christiansen, MSN, RN
Professor, Associate Degree Nursing
Tyler Junior College
Tyler, Texas

M. Kathleen Dwinnells, MSN, RNC, CNS
Assistant Professor of Nursing
Kent State University at Trumbull
Warren, Ohio

Susan Estes-Blakey, RN, MSN
Assistant Professor
Georgia Baptist College of Nursing of Mercer University
Atlanta, Georgia

Debra Ferguson, RN, MSN
Instructor
Gadsden State Community College
Gadsden, Alabama

Audrey N. Jones, RN, MSN
Nurse Faculty
Jefferson State Community College
Birmingham, Alabama

Kathy J. Keister, PHD, RN, CNE
Associate Professor
Wright State University
College of Nursing & Health
Dayton, Ohio

Lori Kulju, MSN, RN
Assistant Professor
Bellin College
Green Bay, Wisconsin

Kelli Lewis
Rend Lake College
Ina, Illinois

Laura Burgess Patton, RN, MN
Professor of Nursing
Gordon College
Barnesville, Georgia

Lisa Richwine
Ivy Tech Community College
Anderson, Indiana

Laura R. Romero, RN, MSN, CNM
Retired Nursing Instructor
East Los Angeles College
Monterey Park, California

Lynda Shand
College of New Rochelle
New Rochelle, New York

Koreen W. Smiley, RN, MSN, MSEd
Nursing Professor
St. Charles Community College
Cottleville, Missouri

Sherri L. Smith, RN
Practical Nursing Program Chairman
Arkansas State University Technical Center
Jonesboro, Arkansas

Lisa Soontupe, EdD, RN
Associate Professor
Nova Southeastern University
Fort Lauderdale, Florida

Lee Ann Waltz
University of the Incarnate Word
San Antonio, Texas

Melinda Wang
Roane State Community College
Knoxville, Tennessee

Preface

*T*he idea for this compact, pocket-sized book about dosage calculation was generated by my students. For several years I watched as they took their math-related handouts and photocopied them, reducing them to a size that would fit into the pockets of their uniforms or laboratory coats. This "pocket" reference material was readily accessible when a math calculation was needed to administer a drug. Each year the number of papers that were copied increased as each group of students passed on their ideas to the next group. I also noted that staff nurses were using this readily available and compact information as a reference for math problems.

When a student asked, "Why not put together for us all the information that we need?" I thought, "Why not?" The idea was born, the commitment made, and 18 months later the first edition of *Math for Nurses* was published in 1987. It is my hope that it will continue, in this eighth edition, to be helpful to all who need a quick reference source when struggling with dosage calculations and drug preparation.

How to Use This Book

This book is designed for two purposes:

- To help you learn how to quickly and accurately calculate drug dosages and administer medications.
- To serve as a quick reference when reinforcement of learning is required.

The best way to use this pocket guide is to:

- Read the rules and examples.
- Follow the steps for solving the problems.
- Work the practice problems.
- Write down your answers and notes in the margin so that you have a quick reference when you need to review.

Organization

This pocket guide is divided into three units to facilitate quick access to specific information needed to administer drugs. The preassessment test should be completed before beginning. Unit 1 presents a review of basic math. Chapters 2 and 3 cover common fractions and decimals. Chapter 4 shows how to set up a ratio and proportion and solve for x, using a colon or fraction format. Drug-related word problems are used as contemporary examples. This unit information is essential, forming a foundation for understanding the complex dosage calculations presented in Unit 3.

Unit 2 explains measurement systems. The metric system, the apothecary system, and household units of measurement are given in Chapter 5. Emphasis on the apothecary system has been limited because of the need to minimize use of the system. Chapter 6 presents approximate system equivalents and shows how to convert from one unit of measurement to another. Some of these system equivalents are duplicated on the insert card, to provide quick and easy access when calculating drug dosage problems.

Unit 3, Dosage Calculations, is the most comprehensive and detailed section of this pocket guide. The unit begins with a detailed description of how to read and interpret medication labels in Chapter 7. Sample dosage questions specific to a drug label are used as examples. Chapters 8 and 9 cover oral and parenteral dosage calculations. Ratio and proportion and the Formula Method are used for every problem. Dimensional analysis, presented in detail in Chapter 8, is also incorporated into every drug calculation. The intravenous therapy content has been expanded in Chapter 10. Critical care applications have also been expanded in Chapter 11. The last four chapters incorporate intravenous insulin (Chapter 12), weight-based heparin (Chapter 13), intravenous (IV) push medications for children (Chapter 14), and expanded examples of drug reconstitution (Chapter 15). Throughout this unit, problem-solving methodology is presented in a simple, easy-to-follow manner. A step-by-step approach is used, which will guide the reader through each set of examples. Enrichment information can be found in the appendices.

Special Features

A **pocket-size laminated insert card** containing approximate system equivalents and conversion formulas is included for quick and easy access when calculating drug dosage problems. This popular feature has been retained in this edition, along with the **Critical Thinking Checks**—questions designed to help you analyze the results of your answer to a dosage problem. They appear frequently throughout the book.

New Content in This Edition

- **Practice Problems on thePoint.** In an effort to maintain the size of the book yet meet the student and faculty requests for more questions, 300 new practice problems have been put online. Throughout the chapters, you will be referred to http://thePoint.lww.com/Boyer8e to access these additional questions. Use the code in the front of your book to access these online practice problems. Answer Keys are available to check your work.
- **Dimensional analysis (DA)** has been expanded in Chapter 8 to show the different ways that the formula can be used. This method is used consistently throughout the book, along with ratio and proportion and the Formula Method, as one of three ways to calculate dosages.
- **Learning objectives** have been expanded in every chapter to help guide you in your learning.
- The reference **insert card** has been updated with dosage calculation formulas, and the content related to apothecary equivalents has been decreased.
- **Pictures, charts, and tables** have been updated.
- New content has been added for IV push medications, including pediatric considerations.

Revised and Expanded Chapters

- Chapter 5: The Metric, Household, and Apothecary Systems of Measurement

Math for Nurses was written for all nurses who administer drugs. It is intended as a quick, easy, and readily accessible guide when dosage calculations are required. It is my hope that its use will help nurses to calculate dosages accurately and, as a result, to improve the accuracy of drug delivery. As you use this book, please email me at mboyer@dccc.edu with your comments and/or suggestions for improvement.

It is our inherent responsibility as nurses to ensure that every patient entrusted to our care receives the correct dosage of medication delivered in the most appropriate way.

Mary Jo Boyer, RN, PhD

Contents

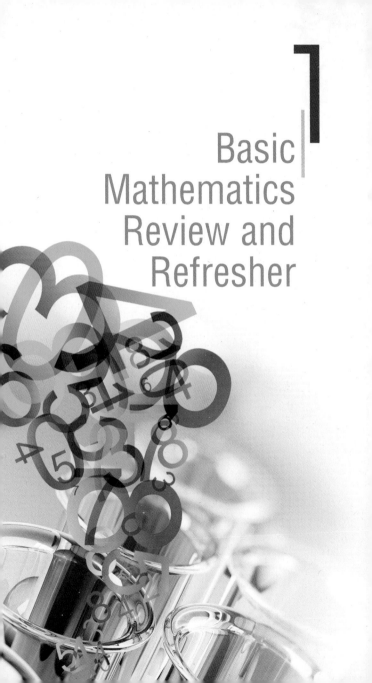

Basic Mathematics Review and Refresher

1

*T*his unit presents a basic review of fractions, decimals, percents, and ratio-proportion. The ability to solve for *x* assumes a basic mastery of fractions and decimals. Therefore, a brief discussion of addition, subtraction, multiplication, and division for fractions and decimals is provided in Chapters 2 and 3 so you can review this material. In order to accurately calculate dosage problems, you need to be able to transcribe a word problem into a mathematical equation. This process is presented in a step-by-step format in Chapter 4. An end-of-unit review is provided to reinforce the rules.

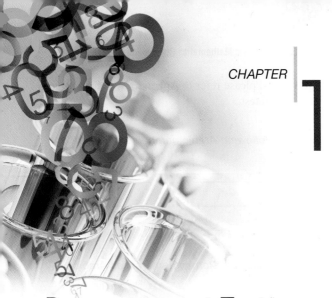

Preassessment Test:
MATHEMATICS SKILLS REVIEW

*B*asic math skills are needed to calculate most dosage and solution problems encountered in clinical practice. This pretest will help you understand your ability to solve fraction, decimal, and percentage problems and determine the value of an unknown (*x*) using the ratio-proportion.

There are 100 questions, each worth one point. Answers are listed in the back of the book. A score of 90% or greater means that you have mastered the knowledge necessary to proceed directly to Unit II. Begin by setting aside 1 hour. You will need scrap paper. Take time to work out your answers and avoid careless mistakes. If an answer is incorrect, please review the corresponding section in Unit I. If you need to review Roman numerals and associated Arabic equivalents, please refer to Appendix A before beginning the pretest.

Write the following Arabic numbers as Roman numerals.

1. 8 _____   2. 13 _____

3. 10 _____   4. 37 _____

5. 51 _____

Write the following Roman numerals as Arabic numbers.

6. xv _____   7. xvi _____

8. LXV _____   9. ix _____

10. xix _____

Add or subtract the following fractions. Reduce to lowest terms.

11. $\dfrac{1}{2} + \dfrac{1}{8} =$ _____   12. $\dfrac{3}{4} - \dfrac{1}{4} =$ _____

13. $\dfrac{1}{5} + \dfrac{3}{10} =$ _____   14. $\dfrac{4}{6} - \dfrac{2}{5} =$ _____

Choose the fraction that has the largest value.

15. $\dfrac{1}{3}$ or $\dfrac{1}{6}$ _____   16. $\dfrac{1}{150}$ or $\dfrac{1}{200}$ _____

17. $\dfrac{1}{100}$ or $\dfrac{1}{150}$ _____   18. $\dfrac{1}{2}$ or $\dfrac{3}{4}$ _____

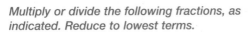

Multiply or divide the following fractions, as indicated. Reduce to lowest terms.

19. $\dfrac{1}{2} \times \dfrac{3}{4} =$ _____   20. $2\dfrac{2}{5} \times 3\dfrac{5}{10} =$ _____

21. $\dfrac{1}{4} \div \dfrac{1}{3} =$ _____   22. $3\dfrac{1}{2} \div \dfrac{4}{7} =$ _____

23. $\dfrac{1}{150} \times 2\dfrac{1}{2} =$ _____   24. $\dfrac{8}{7} \times 3 =$ _____

25. $\dfrac{1}{8} \div 6 =$ _____   26. $4\dfrac{2}{5} \div 11 =$ _____

Change the following mixed numbers to improper fractions.

27. $2\dfrac{4}{5}$ _____   28. $6\dfrac{3}{4}$ _____

29. $10\dfrac{4}{9}$ _____   30. $8\dfrac{1}{7}$ _____

Change these improper fractions to whole or mixed numbers. Reduce to lowest terms.

31. $\dfrac{120}{40}$ _____   32. $\dfrac{146}{36}$ _____

33. $\dfrac{35}{11}$ _____   34. $\dfrac{16}{13}$ _____

Change the following fractions to decimals. Remember to place a 0 before the decimal point when the decimal is less than (<) one.

35. $\dfrac{1}{3}$ _____   36. $\dfrac{2}{5}$ _____

37. $\dfrac{3}{8}$ _____ 38. $\dfrac{3}{4}$ _____

Add or subtract the following decimals, as indicated.

39. $0.36 + 1.45 =$ _____

40. $3.71 + 0.29 =$ _____

41. $6 - 0.13 =$ _____

42. $2.14 - 0.01 =$ _____

Multiply or divide the following decimals, as indicated.

43. $6 \times 8.13 =$ _____

44. $0.125 \times 2 =$ _____

45. $21.6 \div 0.3 =$ _____

46. $7.82 \div 2.3 =$ _____

Change the following decimals to fractions. Reduce to lowest terms.

47. 0.25 _____   48. 0.80 _____

49. 0.33 _____   50. 0.45 _____

51. 0.75 _____   52. 0.60 _____

Solve for the value of x in the following ratio and proportion problems.

53. $4.2 : 14 :: x : 10$ _____

54. $0.8 : 4 :: 3.2 : x$ _____

55. $6 : 2 :: 8 : x$ _____

56. $5 : 20 :: x : 40$ _____

57. $0.25 : 200 :: x : 600$ _____

58. $\frac{1}{5} : x :: \frac{1}{20} : 3$ _____

59. $12 : x :: 8 : 16$ _____

60. $x : \frac{4}{5} :: 0.60 : 3$ _____

61. $0.3 : 12 :: x : 36$ _____

62. $x : 8 :: \frac{1}{4} : 10$ _____

Change the following fractions and decimals to percentages.

63. $\frac{1}{5}$ _____   64. 0.36 _____

65. 0.07 _____   66. $\frac{5}{40}$ _____

67. 0.103 _____   68. 1.83 _____

69. $\frac{4}{16}$ _____   70. $60/100$ _____

71. 0.01 _____   72. 1.98 _____

73. $\frac{120}{100}$ _____   74. $\frac{8}{56}$ _____

Change the following percents to decimals.

75. 25% _____   76. 40% _____

77. 80% _____   78. 15% _____

79. 4.8% _____   80. 0.36% _____

81. 1.75% _____   82. 8.30% _____

Solve the following percent equations.

83. 30% of 60 _____

84. 4.5% of 200 _____

85. 0.6% of 180 _____

86. 30 is 75% of _____

87. 20 is 80% of _____

88. What % of 80 is 20? _____

89. What % of 60 is 12? _____

90. What % of 72 is 18? _____

91. 15 is 30% of _____

92. 60 is 50% of _____

Write each of the following measures in its related equivalency. Reduce to lowest terms.

	Percent	Colon Ratio	Common Fractions	Decimal
93.	25%	_____	_____	_____
94.	_____	1 : 30	_____	_____
95.	_____	_____	_____	0.05
96.	_____	_____	$\frac{1}{150}$	_____
97.	0.45%	_____	_____	_____
98.	_____	1 : 100	_____	_____
99.	_____	_____	$\frac{1}{120}$	_____
100.	_____	_____	_____	0.50

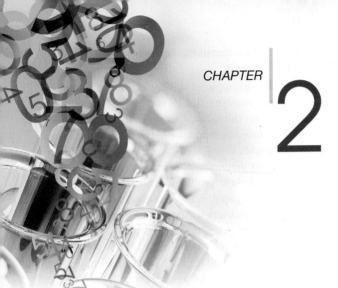

Fractions

LEARNING OBJECTIVES

After completing this chapter, you should be able to:

- Understand the concept of a fraction—the number of parts to a whole.
- Distinguish between the four types of fractions, the concept of size, and the fraction value relative to the value of one (1).
- Convert fractions and reduce them to their lowest terms.
- Add, subtract, multiply, and divide fractions.

*T*he term *fraction* means a type of division. A *fraction* is a part or piece of a whole number that *indicates division of that number into equal units or parts.* A fraction is written with one number over another, for example, 1/4, 2/5; therefore, the line between the numbers is a *division sign*. The number *above the line (numerator)* is divided by the number *under the line (denominator)*. Because the fraction (1/4) represents division, it can be read as numerator (1) divided by denominator (4). You need to know how to calculate dosage problems with fractions because they are used in apothecary and household measures, as well as in a variety of reports, medical orders, and documents used in health care.

Look at the circles in Figure 2.1. They are divided into equal parts (4 and 8). Each part of the circle (1) is a fraction or piece of the whole (1/4 or 1/8).

The Denominator of a Fraction

The denominator of a fraction refers to the total number of equal parts into which the whole has been divided. If you divide a circle into four equal parts, the *total number of parts* (4) that you are working with is the *bottom* number of the fraction and is called the *denominator*. If you divide the circle into eight equal parts, the denominator is 8. The denominator is also called the *divisor*.

_R U L E_

The denominator refers to the *total number of equal parts* and is the number on the bottom of the fraction. The larger the number in the denominator, the smaller the value of the equal parts (or fraction) of the whole. See Figure 2.1.

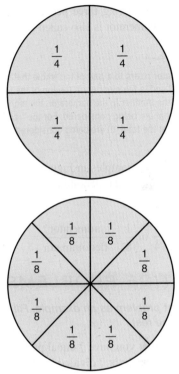

FIGURE 2.1 Two circles: the whole divided into equal parts.

The Numerator of a Fraction

The numerator of a fraction tells you how many parts of the whole are being considered. If you divide a circle into four equal parts, each part (1) that you are considering is the *top* number of the fraction and is called the *numerator*. If you divide the circle into eight equal parts,

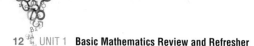
and you are considering three parts, the numerator is three (3). The numerator is also called the *dividend*.

RULE

The numerator refers to a *part* of the whole that is being considered and is the number on the top of the fraction. The larger the number in the numerator, the more parts of the whole that are being considered. For the fraction 3/8, three parts of the total (8) are being considered.

In the circle examples in Figure 2.1, the numerator in both is 1 and the denominator is either 4 or 8. Therefore,

$$\text{Fraction} = \frac{1}{4} \text{ or } \frac{1}{8} = \frac{\text{numerator}}{\text{denominator}} = \text{"divided by"}$$

PRACTICE PROBLEMS

Use the first problem as an example. Fill in the blanks for the rest.

1. 7/8 means that you have <u>7</u> equal parts, each worth ⅛. The numerator is <u>7</u> divided by the denominator, which is <u>8</u>.

2. 9/10 means that you have _____ equal parts, each worth _____. The denominator is _____.

3. 4/5 means that you have _____ equal parts, each worth _____. The numerator is _____ divided by the denominator, which is _____.

4. 3/4 means that you have _____ equal parts, each worth _____. The denominator is _____.

Concept of Size

RULE

When the numerators are the same, the larger the number in the denominator, the *smaller the value of the parts* (or fraction) of the whole.

Look at Figure 2.1, which illustrates two circles: one is divided into fourths, and one is divided into eighths. As you look at the circles, you will notice that the circle that is divided into eighths has smaller portions than the circle that is divided into fourths. The reason is that the value of each part of the fraction 1/8 is less than the value of each part of the fraction 1/4. Even though 1/8 has a larger denominator (8) than does 1/4 (4), it is a smaller fraction. This is an important concept to understand; that is, the larger the number or value in the denominator, the smaller the fraction or parts of the whole. For example:

$$\frac{1}{2} \text{ is larger than } \frac{1}{4}$$

$$\frac{1}{8} \text{ is larger than } \frac{1}{16}$$

$$\frac{1}{9} \text{ is larger than } \frac{1}{10}$$

RULE

When the denominators are the same, the larger the number in the numerator, the *larger the value of the parts* of the whole.

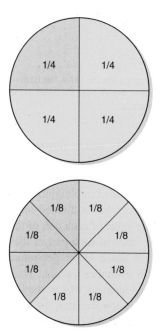

FIGURE 2.2 Two circles: shaded areas indicate larger sizes.

Look at Figure 2.2. The shaded area in the top circle shows that 3/4 is larger than 1/4. The shaded area in the bottom circle shows that 5/8 is larger than 3/8.

PRACTICE PROBLEMS

Indicate which fractions are larger.

1. 1/2 or 1/4 _____   2. 1/8 or 1/16 _____

3. 1/9 or 1/10 _____   4. 2/5 or 4/5 _____

5. 1/6 or 4/6 _____   6. 3/15 or 8/15 _____

Arrange the following fractions in order of size. That is, list the fraction with the smallest value first, then the next larger fraction, and so on until you end with the largest-valued fraction last.

$$\frac{1}{9} \quad \frac{1}{12} \quad \frac{1}{3} \quad \frac{1}{7} \quad \frac{1}{150} \quad \frac{1}{25} \quad \frac{1}{100} \quad \frac{1}{300} \quad \frac{1}{75}$$

Types of Fractions and Value

Fractions That Are Less Than One (<1), Equal to One (1), and Greater Than One (>1)

Common fractions can be divided into four groups: *proper* fractions, *improper* fractions, *mixed numbers*, and *complex fractions*.

___R U L E___

If the numerator is *less than* the denominator, the fraction value is *less than one.* These fractions are called *proper fractions.*

EXAMPLES: $\dfrac{3}{4} < 1, \quad \dfrac{7}{8} < 1, \quad \dfrac{9}{10} < 1$

___R U L E___

If the numerator and denominator are *equal to each other,* the fraction value is *equal to one.* These fractions are called *improper fractions.*

EXAMPLES: $\dfrac{1}{1} = 1, \quad \dfrac{3}{3} = 1, \quad \dfrac{25}{25} = 1$

RULE

If the numerator is *greater than* the denominator, the fraction value is *greater than one*. These fractions are also called *improper* fractions.

EXAMPLES: $\dfrac{2}{1} = 2 > 1, \quad \dfrac{5}{4} = 1\dfrac{1}{4} > 1$

RULE

If a fraction and a whole number are *written together*, the fraction value is *always greater than one*. These fractions are *mixed* numbers.

EXAMPLES: $1\dfrac{1}{2} > 1, \quad 3\dfrac{3}{4} > 1, \quad 5\dfrac{4}{5} > 1$

RULE

If a fraction includes a combination of whole numbers and proper and improper fractions in both the numerator and the denominator, the value may be *less than, equal to,* or *greater than one*. These fractions are called *complex* fractions.

EXAMPLES: $\dfrac{\frac{1}{2}}{2} < 1, \quad \dfrac{\frac{3}{12}}{\frac{5}{20}} = 1, \quad \dfrac{\frac{8}{14}}{\frac{1}{3}} > 1$

Equivalent or Equal Fractions

Change Fractions to Equivalent or Equal Fractions

When you are working problems with fractions, it is sometimes necessary to change a fraction to a different but equivalent fraction to make the math problem easier to calculate. For example, it may be necessary to change 2/4 to 1/2 or 2/3 to 4/6. You can make a new fraction that has the same value by either multiplying or dividing *both the numerator and the denominator by the same number.* Look at the following examples.

EXAMPLES: $\dfrac{2}{3}$ can be changed to $\dfrac{4}{6}$ by multiplying both the numerator and the denominator by 2.

$$\left(\dfrac{2 \times 2 = 4}{3 \times 2 = 6} \right)$$

$\dfrac{2}{4}$ can be changed to $\dfrac{1}{2}$ by dividing both the numerator and the denominator by 2.

$$\left(\dfrac{2 \div 2 = 1}{4 \div 2 = 2} \right)$$

It is important to remember that you can change the numerator and the denominator of a fraction and the value of the fraction will be unchanged *as long as you follow the following rule:*

RULE

When changing a fraction yet keeping the same equivalent value, you must do the same thing (multiply or divide by the same number) to the numerator and to the denominator.

EXAMPLES: To change the fraction $\frac{4}{5}$ to $\frac{8}{10}$, multiply 4×2 and 5×2.

$$\left(\begin{array}{l} 4 \times 2 = 8 \\ 5 \times 2 = 10 \end{array}\right)$$

$\frac{4}{5}$ has the same value as $\frac{8}{10}$.

To change the fraction $\frac{4}{16}$ to $\frac{1}{4}$, divide 4 by 4 and 16 by 4.

$$\left(\begin{array}{l} 4 \div 4 = 1 \\ 16 \div 4 = 4 \end{array}\right)$$

To determine that both fractions have equal value, multiply the opposite numerators and denominators. For example, if 4/5 = 8/10, then the product of 4×10 will equal the product of 5×8.

$$4 \times 10 = 40 \quad \text{and} \quad 5 \times 8 = 40$$

PRACTICE PROBLEMS

Circle the correct answer.

1. 3/5 is equivalent to: 6/15 or 9/10 or 12/20

2. 4/8 is equivalent to: 8/24 or 12/16 or 20/40

3. 6/12 is equivalent to: 2/4 or 3/5 or 12/36

4. 10/16 is equivalent to: 20/48 or 5/8 or 30/32

5. 12/20 is equivalent to: 3/5 or 6/5 or 4/10

6. 18/30 is equivalent to: 3/15 or 9/10 or 6/10

7. 9/54 is equivalent to: 3/16 or 1/6 or 1/8

8. 15/90 is equivalent to: 1/6 or 3/8 or 5/14

9. 14/56 is equivalent to: 2/6 or 1/4 or 7/8

10. 8/144 is equivalent to: 2/36 or 4/23 or 1/18

Simplify or Reduce Fractions to Their Lowest Terms

When calculating dosages, it is easier to work with fractions that have been simplified, or reduced to the lowest terms. This means that the numerator and the denominator are the smallest numbers that can still represent the fraction or piece of the whole. For example, 4/10 can be reduced to 2/5; 4/8 can be reduced to 1/2. It is important to know how to reduce (or simplify) a fraction. The following rule outlines the steps for reducing a fraction to its lowest terms. Remember: You may have to reduce several times.

RULE

To reduce a fraction to its lowest terms: Divide both the numerator and the denominator by the *largest* number that can go evenly into both.

EXAMPLES:	Reduce the fraction $\dfrac{9}{18}$ to its lowest terms.

$$\left(\frac{9 \div 9 = 1}{18 \div 9 = 2} \right)$$

The largest number that can be used to divide *both* the numerator (9) and the denominator (18) is 9.

Reduce: $\dfrac{6}{10}$ can be reduced to $\dfrac{3}{5}$ by dividing both the numerator and the denominator by 2.

Reduce: $\dfrac{33}{132}$ can be reduced to $\dfrac{11}{44}$ by dividing both the numerator and the denominator by 3. Then $\dfrac{11}{44}$ can be reduced again to $\dfrac{1}{4}$ by dividing by 11.

PRACTICE PROBLEMS

Reduce the following fractions to their lowest terms:

1. $\dfrac{8}{48}$ _____ 2. $\dfrac{6}{36}$ _____ 3. $\dfrac{2}{18}$ _____ 4. $\dfrac{10}{60}$ _____

5. $\dfrac{4}{36}$ _____ 6. $\dfrac{3}{12}$ _____ 7. $\dfrac{35}{105}$ _____ 8. $\dfrac{63}{105}$ _____

Find the Least Common Denominator

_R U L E_

To find the least common denominator (LCD): Find the _smallest_ number that is easily divided by both denominators and then change the fraction to equivalent fractions, each with the same denominator. Remember: least common denominator = smallest number.

When beginning, first see if any of the denominators can be easily divided by each of the other denominators. If so, that number now becomes your new LCD.

EXAMPLE: Add $\dfrac{1}{4} + \dfrac{3}{5}$

- Find the _smallest_ number (LCD) that all the denominators can be divided evenly into.

$$\dfrac{1}{4} + \dfrac{3}{5} \qquad \text{The LCD} = 20$$

- Change the unlike fractions to equivalent or equal fractions using the LCD. Divide the LCD by the denominator and then multiply that number by the numerator.

$$\dfrac{1}{4} = \dfrac{5}{20} \qquad \dfrac{3}{5} = \dfrac{12}{20}$$

- Add the new numerators and place that number over the new LCD.

$$\dfrac{5}{20} + \dfrac{12}{20} = \dfrac{17}{20}$$

ANSWER: $\dfrac{17}{20}$

- Reduce and change any improper fraction to a mixed number, if necessary.

EXAMPLE: Add $\dfrac{1}{3} + \dfrac{5}{6}$ The LCD = 6

- Change $\dfrac{1}{3}$ to $\dfrac{2}{6}$ and $\dfrac{5}{6}$ stays $\dfrac{5}{6}$

- Add the new numerators and place that number over the new LCD.

$$2 + 5 = 7\,\dfrac{7}{6}$$

- Change the improper fraction to a mixed number.

$$\dfrac{7}{6} \text{ is changed to } 1\dfrac{1}{6}$$

ANSWER: $1\dfrac{1}{6}$

Conversion

Convert Mixed Numbers and Improper Fractions

You need to know how to convert a variety of fractions to make drug dosage calculations easier. A mixed number (1 1/4) can be changed to an improper fraction (5/4) and an improper fraction (3/2) can be changed to a mixed number (1 1/2). If you get a final answer that is an improper fraction, convert it to a mixed number. For example, it is better to say "I have 1 1/4 apples" than to say "I have 5/4 apples."

To understand how to convert fractions, follow these rules.

Change a Mixed Number to an Improper Fraction

RULE

To change a mixed number to an improper fraction: Multiply the denominator by the whole number and then add the numerator to that sum.

EXAMPLE: Change $2\dfrac{3}{4}$ to an improper fraction.

$$2\frac{3}{4} = 4 \times 2 = 8 \qquad 8 + 3 = 11$$

The answer (11) becomes the *new numerator* of the new single fraction. The denominator in the original stays the same.

$$2\frac{3}{4} = \frac{11}{4}$$

The *mixed number* $2\dfrac{3}{4}$ becomes the *improper fraction* $\dfrac{11}{4}$.

PRACTICE PROBLEMS

Change the following mixed numbers to improper fractions:

1. $5\dfrac{9}{12}$ _____   2. $6\dfrac{7}{8}$ _____

3. $8\dfrac{3}{5}$ _____   4. $15\dfrac{1}{9}$ _____

5. $32\dfrac{2}{3}$ _____   6. $21\dfrac{3}{4}$ _____

7. $18\dfrac{1}{2}$ _____   8. $6\dfrac{3}{9}$ _____

9. $5\dfrac{2}{5}$ _____   10. $11\dfrac{1}{6}$ _____

Change an Improper Fraction to a Mixed Number

RULE

To change an improper fraction to a mixed or whole number: Divide the numerator by the denominator and then use the leftover numbers as the new numerator and the new denominator of the mixed number. The quotient becomes the whole number of the mixed number.

EXAMPLE: Change $\dfrac{13}{7}$ to a mixed number.

The number that you get (1) when you divide the numerator (13) by the denominator (7) becomes the whole number of the mixed number.

$13 \div 7 = 1$ (new whole number)

The *remainder,* or number that you have left over (6), becomes the numerator of the fraction that goes with the whole number to make it a mixed number.

$$13 \div 7 = 1\dfrac{6}{?}$$

The *original* denominator of the improper fraction (7) becomes the denominator of the fraction of the mixed number.

$$13 \div 7 = 1\dfrac{6}{7}$$

Any remainder is reduced to the lowest terms.

ANSWER: $1\dfrac{6}{7}$

PRACTICE PROBLEMS

Change the following improper fractions to mixed numbers:

1. $\dfrac{30}{4}$ _____

2. $\dfrac{41}{6}$ _____

3. $\dfrac{68}{9}$ _____

4. $\dfrac{72}{11}$ _____

5. $\dfrac{90}{12}$ _____

6. $\dfrac{40}{15}$ _____

7. $\dfrac{86}{20}$ _____

8. $\dfrac{62}{8}$ _____

9. $\dfrac{86}{9}$ _____

10. $\dfrac{112}{6}$ _____

Addition of Fractions

When fractions are added, *no calculations are done on the denominators*; only the numerators are added. Therefore, fractions can be added *only when the denominators are the same*. Denominators that are different (unlike) must be made the same.

Add Fractions When the Denominators Are the Same

RULE

To add fractions with the same denominators: Add the numerators and place the new sum over the similar denominator. Reduce to lowest terms and change to a mixed number if necessary.

EXAMPLE: Add $\dfrac{1}{5} + \dfrac{3}{5}$

- Add the numerators. For example:

$$\frac{1}{5} + \frac{3}{5} = \frac{1+3}{} = 4$$

- Place the new sum over the same denominator.

$$\frac{1}{5} + \frac{3}{5} = \frac{4}{5} = \frac{\text{new numerator}}{\text{same denominator}}$$

ANSWER: $\frac{4}{5}$

EXAMPLE: Add $\frac{1}{7} + \frac{4}{7}$

Change: $\frac{1}{7} + \frac{4}{7} = \frac{1+4}{} = \frac{5}{7}$

$\frac{5}{} = $ new numerator

$\frac{}{7} = $ same denominator

ANSWER: $\frac{5}{7}$

EXAMPLE: Add $\frac{1}{6} + \frac{9}{6}$

Change: $\frac{1}{6} + \frac{9}{6} = \frac{1+9}{} = \frac{10}{6}$

$\frac{10}{} = $ new numerator

$\frac{}{6} = $ same denominator

$\frac{10}{6}$ need to be reduced

Reduce: $\dfrac{10}{6} = \dfrac{10 \div 2}{6 \div 2} = \dfrac{5}{3} =$ improper fraction

Change: $\dfrac{5}{3} = 5 \div 3 = 1\dfrac{2}{3} =$ a mixed number

ANSWER: $1\dfrac{2}{3}$

Add Fractions When the Denominators Are Not the Same

_R U L E_

To add fractions when the denominators are not the same: Find the least common denominator (LCD) of each fraction, take each new quotient and multiply it by each numerator, add the numerators, place the new sum over the LCD, and reduce to lowest terms.

EXAMPLE: Add $\dfrac{1}{4} + \dfrac{3}{5}$ The LCD is 20

- Divide the LCD of 20 by the denominator of each fraction to get the new *quotient*.

$$\frac{1}{4} = \frac{}{20} \qquad 20 \div 4 = 5$$

$$\frac{3}{5} = \frac{}{20} \qquad 20 \div 5 = 4$$

- Take each new quotient and multiply it by the numerator of each fraction.

$$5 \text{ (new quotient)} \times 1 \text{ (numerator)} = \frac{5}{20}$$

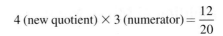

$$4 \text{ (new quotient)} \times 3 \text{ (numerator)} = \frac{12}{20}$$

- Add the new numerators. Place the new sum over the LCD. Reduce to lowest terms.

$$\frac{5}{20} + \frac{12}{20} = \frac{17}{20}$$

ANSWER: $\dfrac{17}{20}$

EXAMPLE: Add $\dfrac{1}{3} + \dfrac{5}{6}$

The LCD is 6.

$$\frac{1}{3} = \frac{}{6} \qquad 6 \div 3 = 2 \times 1 = 2$$

$$\frac{5}{6} = \frac{}{6} \qquad 6 \div 6 = 1 \times 5 = 5$$

- Add the new numerators.

$$\frac{2}{6} + \frac{5}{6} = \frac{2+5}{6} = \frac{7}{6}$$

- Change any improper fraction to a mixed number.

$$\frac{7}{6} \text{ should be changed to } 1\frac{1}{6}.$$

ANSWER: $1\dfrac{1}{6}$

Addition of Mixed Numbers

R U L E

To add fractions with a mixed number: Change any mixed number to an improper fraction, find the LCD, change to similar fractions, add the new numerators, and reduce to lowest terms.

EXAMPLE: Add $\dfrac{1}{6} + 2\dfrac{3}{8} + \dfrac{5}{6}$

- Change the mixed number to an improper fraction.

$$2\dfrac{3}{8} \text{ becomes } \dfrac{19}{8}$$

- Find the LCD. For the denominators of 6 and 8, use the LCD of 24.

- Change the different fractions to fractions with the same denominator.

$$\dfrac{1}{6} \text{ becomes } \dfrac{4}{24}$$

$$\dfrac{19}{8} \text{ becomes } \dfrac{57}{24}$$

$$\dfrac{5}{6} \text{ becomes } \dfrac{20}{24}$$

- Add the new numerators and place your answer over the LCD.

$$\dfrac{4 + 57 + 20}{} = \dfrac{81}{24}$$

- Reduce to lowest terms and change to a mixed number.

$$\frac{81}{24} = \frac{27}{8} = 3\frac{3}{8}$$

ANSWER: $3\frac{3}{8}$

Subtraction of Fractions

Fractions can be subtracted *only when the denominators are the same* because only the numerators are subtracted. Denominators that are unlike must be made the same.

Subtract Fractions When the Denominators Are the Same

RULE

To subtract fractions when the denominators are the same, *only subtract the numerators.* Reduce to lowest terms.

| EXAMPLE: Subtract $\frac{5}{6} - \frac{3}{6}$

- Subtract $\frac{5}{6} - \frac{3}{6} = \frac{5-3}{6} = \frac{2}{6}$

- Reduce $\frac{2}{6} = \frac{1}{3}$, a new fraction

ANSWER: $\frac{1}{3}$

EXAMPLE: Subtract $\dfrac{7}{8} - \dfrac{4}{8} = \dfrac{7-4}{} = \dfrac{3}{8}$

$\dfrac{3}{8}$, a new fraction

ANSWER: $\dfrac{3}{8}$

EXAMPLE: Subtract $\dfrac{7}{8} - \dfrac{3}{8} = \dfrac{4}{8}$

• Reduce $\dfrac{4}{8} = \dfrac{1}{2}$, a new fraction

ANSWER: $\dfrac{1}{2}$

Subtract Fractions When the Denominators Are Not the Same

You will probably never need to subtract fractions with different denominators or fractions with a mixed number to calculate dosage problems. However, both will be presented here briefly just in case the situation occurs.

RULE

To subtract fractions when the denominators are not the same: Find the LCD, change to similar fractions, and subtract the new numerators. Reduce to lowest terms.

EXAMPLE: Subtract $\dfrac{5}{6} - \dfrac{3}{5}$

• Find the least common denominator.

$$\dfrac{5}{6} - \dfrac{3}{5} = 30 \text{ (LCD)}$$

- Change to similar or equal fractions. Refer back to pages 21–26.

$$\frac{5}{6} \text{ becomes } \frac{25}{30}$$

$$\frac{3}{5} \text{ becomes } \frac{18}{30}$$

- Subtract the new numerators and place your answer over the common denominator:

$$\frac{25}{30} - \frac{18}{30} = \frac{25 - 18}{30} = \frac{7}{30}$$

Answer: $\dfrac{7}{30}$

Subtraction of Mixed Numbers

There are two ways to subtract fractions with mixed numbers:

Change the mixed number to an improper fraction or leave the mixed number as a mixed number.

R U L E

To subtract fractions with a mixed number: Change the mixed number to an improper fraction, find the LCD, change to similar fractions, subtract the new numerators, and reduce to lowest terms.

EXAMPLE:

Subtract $2\dfrac{1}{8} - \dfrac{3}{6}$

$$2\dfrac{1}{8} = \dfrac{17}{8} - \dfrac{3}{6}$$

- Find the LCD. For the denominators 8 and 6, use the LCD of 24.

- Change to similar or equal fractions.

$$\dfrac{17}{8} \text{ becomes } \dfrac{51}{24}$$

$$\dfrac{3}{6} \text{ becomes } \dfrac{12}{24}$$

- Subtract the new numerators and place your answer over the common denominator:

$$\dfrac{51}{24} - \dfrac{12}{24} = \dfrac{51-12}{24} = \dfrac{39}{24}$$

- Reduce and change to a mixed number, if necessary.

$$\dfrac{39}{24} \text{ becomes } \dfrac{13}{8} = 1\dfrac{5}{8}$$

ANSWER: $1\dfrac{5}{8}$

RULE

To subtract fractions with a mixed number: Leave the fraction as a mixed number, find the LCD, change to the same denominator, subtract the numerators and the whole number, and reduce to lowest terms.

EXAMPLE: Subtract $2\dfrac{1}{8} - \dfrac{3}{6}$

- Find the LCD. For the denominators of 6 and 8, use the LCD of 24.

$$2\dfrac{1}{8} \text{ becomes } 2\dfrac{3}{24}$$

$$\dfrac{3}{6} \text{ becomes } \dfrac{12}{24}$$

- First, subtract the numerators. Then subtract the whole numbers.

Note: To subtract the larger number (12) from the smaller number (3), you need to borrow 1, or 24/24, from the whole number 2. Then add $24 + 3 = 27$, a new numerator. You can now subtract the smaller number (12) from the larger number (27).

$$2\dfrac{3}{24} = 1\dfrac{27}{24}$$

$$-\dfrac{12}{24} = -\dfrac{12}{24}$$

$$\dfrac{}{} \qquad 1\dfrac{15}{24} = 1\dfrac{5}{8}$$

ANSWER: $1\dfrac{5}{8}$

PRACTICE PROBLEMS

Add and reduce.

1. $\dfrac{5}{11} + \dfrac{9}{11} + \dfrac{13}{11} =$ _____

2. $\dfrac{7}{16} + \dfrac{3}{8} =$ _____

3. $\dfrac{4}{6} + 3\dfrac{1}{8} =$ _____

4. $\dfrac{11}{15} + \dfrac{14}{45} =$ _____

5. $\dfrac{5}{20} + \dfrac{8}{20} + \dfrac{13}{20} =$ _____

6. $\dfrac{9}{19} + 1 =$ _____

7. $\dfrac{4}{7} + \dfrac{9}{14} =$ _____

8. $10 + \dfrac{1}{9} + \dfrac{2}{5} =$ _____

9. $\dfrac{17}{24} + \dfrac{11}{12} =$ _____

10. $\dfrac{4}{5} + \dfrac{1}{10} + \dfrac{2}{3} =$ _____

thePoint Additional practice problems to enhance learning and facilitate chapter comprehension can be found at **http://thePoint.lww.com/Boyer8e**.

Subtract and reduce.

11. $\dfrac{6}{7} - \dfrac{3}{7} =$ _____

12. $\dfrac{8}{9} - \dfrac{4}{9} =$ _____

13. $\dfrac{3}{5} - \dfrac{1}{6} =$ _____

14. $\dfrac{3}{4} - \dfrac{2}{9} =$ _____

15. $6\dfrac{3}{7} - \dfrac{2}{3} =$ _____

16. $3\dfrac{1}{4} - 2\dfrac{1}{6} =$ _____

thePoint. Additional practice problems to enhance learning and facilitate chapter comprehension can be found at **http://thePoint.lww.com/Boyer8e.**

Multiplication of Fractions

Multiply a Fraction by Another Fraction

RULE

To multiply fractions: Multiply the numerators, multiply the denominators, and reduce the product to lowest terms. Reducing can be done before multiplying to make calculations easier. *Remember:* When multiplying a fraction and a whole number, place a one (1) under the whole number so it is expressed as a fraction.

EXAMPLES:

$$\frac{3}{4} \times \frac{2}{3} = \frac{3 \times 2}{4 \times 3} = \frac{6}{12} = \frac{1}{2}$$

$$\frac{1}{2} \times \frac{2}{3} = \frac{1 \times 2}{2 \times 3} = \frac{2}{6} = \frac{1}{3}$$

This method of multiplying fractions is sometimes called the "long form." There is also a "shortcut" method for multiplying fractions, called "cancellation." With cancellation, you simplify the numbers *before* you multiply by reducing the numbers to their lowest terms. The value stays the same. Look at the following example:

EXAMPLE:

$$\frac{1}{4} \times \frac{8}{15}$$

Cancellation can be used because the denominator of the first fraction (4) and the numerator of the second fraction (8) can both be divided by 4 and the value of the fraction does not change. So, if you work the problem, it looks like this:

$$\frac{1}{4} \times \frac{8}{15} = \frac{1}{4_1} \times \frac{8^2}{15}$$

Once you have canceled all the numbers and reduced them to the lowest terms, you can then multiply the new numerators and the new denominators to get your answer.

$$\frac{1}{1} \times \frac{2}{15} = \frac{2}{15}$$

ANSWER: $\frac{2}{15}$

Multiply a Fraction by a Mixed Number

When you multiply a fraction by a mixed number, always change the mixed number to an improper fraction before you work the problem. Remember the following rule.

__R U L E__

To multiply a fraction by a mixed number: Change the mixed number to an improper fraction *before you work the problem.*

EXAMPLE: $1\frac{1}{2} \times \frac{1}{2}$

Change: $1\frac{1}{2}$ to $\frac{3}{2}$

Multiply: $\frac{3}{2} \times \frac{1}{2} = \frac{3}{4}$

ANSWER: $\frac{3}{4}$

EXAMPLE: $1\dfrac{1}{2} \times 4\dfrac{1}{2}$

Change: $1\dfrac{1}{2}$ to $\dfrac{3}{2}$

Change: $4\dfrac{1}{2}$ to $\dfrac{9}{2}$

Multiply: $\dfrac{3}{2} \times \dfrac{9}{2} = \dfrac{27}{4}$ or $6\dfrac{3}{4}$

ANSWER: $6\dfrac{3}{4}$

Division of Fractions

Divide a Fraction by Another Fraction

Sometimes it is necessary to divide fractions in order to calculate a drug dosage. In any problem, the first fraction (dividend) is *divided by* the second fraction (divisor). The divisor is always to the right of the division sign. With division of fractions, the divisor (5/9) is *always inverted* (9/5) to change the math calculation to multiplication! The answer is called the *quotient*. To divide fractions, follow this rule.

RULE

To divide fractions by another fraction: Write your problem as division, invert the divisor, multiply the fractions, and reduce.

EXAMPLE: Divide $\dfrac{4}{5} \div \dfrac{5}{9}$

- Write your problem as division and invert the divisor.

$$\dfrac{4}{5} \text{ (dividend)} \div \dfrac{5}{9} \text{ (divisor)} = \text{quotient}$$

$$\dfrac{4}{5} \times \dfrac{9}{5} \left(\text{inverted } \dfrac{5}{9} \right)$$

- Multiply and reduce. The problem now looks like this:

$$\dfrac{4}{5} \times \dfrac{9}{5} = \dfrac{36}{25} = 1\dfrac{11}{25}$$

ANSWER: $1\dfrac{11}{25}$

EXAMPLE: $\dfrac{7}{8} \div \dfrac{3}{5}$

Invert: $\dfrac{3}{5}$ to $\dfrac{5}{3}$

Multiply: $\dfrac{7}{8} \times \dfrac{5}{3} = \dfrac{35}{24} = 1\dfrac{11}{24}$

ANSWER: $1\dfrac{11}{24}$

Divide a Fraction by a Mixed Number

R U L E

To divide fractions that are mixed numbers: Change the mixed number to an improper fraction and reduce.

EXAMPLE:	$\dfrac{3}{6} \div 1\dfrac{2}{5}$
Change:	$1\dfrac{2}{5}$ to $\dfrac{7}{5}$
Write:	$\dfrac{3}{6} \div \dfrac{7}{5}$
Invert:	$\dfrac{7}{5}$ to $\dfrac{5}{7}$
Multiply:	$\dfrac{3}{6} \times \dfrac{5}{7} = \dfrac{15}{42}$
Reduce:	$\dfrac{15}{42} = \dfrac{5}{14}$

ANSWER: $\dfrac{5}{14}$

PRACTICE PROBLEMS

Multiply and Reduce

1. $\dfrac{8}{15} \times \dfrac{8}{12} =$ _____   2. $\dfrac{5}{9} \times \dfrac{3}{7} =$ _____

3. $\dfrac{6}{16} \times \dfrac{2}{5} =$ _____   4. $2\dfrac{7}{10} \times \dfrac{1}{2} =$ _____

5. $3\dfrac{4}{8} \times \dfrac{3}{16} =$ _____   6. $\dfrac{4}{7} \times \dfrac{10}{11} =$ _____

Divide and Reduce

7. $\dfrac{3}{4} \div \dfrac{1}{9} =$ _____

8. $\dfrac{6}{13} \div \dfrac{2}{5} =$ _____

9. $\dfrac{8}{12} \div \dfrac{3}{7} =$ _____

10. $12 \div \dfrac{1}{3} =$ _____

11. $8\dfrac{7}{10} \div 15 =$ _____

12. $\dfrac{4}{7} \div \dfrac{2}{13} =$ _____

thePoint Additional practice problems to enhance learning and facilitate chapter comprehension can be found at **http://thePoint.lww.com/Boyer8e.**

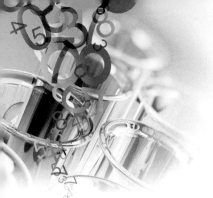

Change the fractions with different denominators to similar fractions by finding the least common denominator:

1. $\dfrac{2}{5}, \dfrac{3}{7}$ _____

2. $\dfrac{7}{5}, \dfrac{4}{20}$ _____

Reduce these fractions to lowest terms:

3. $\dfrac{27}{162} =$ _____

4. $\dfrac{16}{128} =$ _____

Change these improper fractions to mixed numbers:

5. $\dfrac{26}{4} =$ _____

6. $\dfrac{105}{8} =$ _____

Change these mixed numbers to improper fractions:

7. $4\dfrac{6}{11} =$ _____

8. $9\dfrac{2}{23} =$ _____

Reduce these fractions to their lowest terms:

9. $\dfrac{20}{64} =$ _____

10. $\dfrac{16}{128} =$ _____

11. $\dfrac{7}{63} =$ _____   12. $\dfrac{15}{84} =$ _____

Add the following fractions:

13. $\dfrac{1}{9} + \dfrac{7}{9} =$ _____   14. $\dfrac{5}{6} + \dfrac{3}{6} =$ _____

15. $\dfrac{1}{9} + \dfrac{3}{4} =$ _____   16. $6\dfrac{5}{6} + \dfrac{3}{8} =$ _____

Subtract the following fractions:

17. $\dfrac{5}{12} - \dfrac{3}{12} =$ _____   18. $\dfrac{7}{9} - \dfrac{2}{9} =$ _____

19. $\dfrac{3}{4} - \dfrac{1}{6} =$ _____   20. $4\dfrac{6}{10} - \dfrac{3}{8} =$ _____

21. $6\dfrac{3}{8} - 4\dfrac{1}{4} =$ _____   22. $\dfrac{9}{12} - \dfrac{7}{24} =$ _____

Multiply the following fractions:

23. $\dfrac{6}{8} \times \dfrac{1}{5} =$ _____   24. $\dfrac{9}{11} \times \dfrac{1}{3} =$ _____

25. $2\dfrac{1}{10} \times 6\dfrac{6}{9} =$ _____   26. $2\dfrac{2}{7} \times 3\dfrac{4}{8} =$ _____

27. $1\dfrac{5}{11} \times \dfrac{3}{8} =$ _____   28. $\dfrac{4}{3} \times 7\dfrac{2}{4} =$ _____

Divide the following fractions:

29. $\dfrac{3}{5} \div \dfrac{7}{20} =$ _____

30. $\dfrac{8}{9} \div \dfrac{1}{27} =$ _____

31. $6\dfrac{5}{12} \div \dfrac{15}{24} =$ _____

32. $7\dfrac{2}{14} \div 80 =$ _____

33. $16 \div \dfrac{32}{160} =$ _____

34. $4 \div \dfrac{8}{9} =$ _____

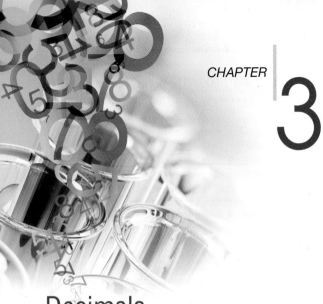

Decimals

LEARNING OBJECTIVES

After completing this chapter, you should be able to:

- Understand the concept of a decimal.
- Read, write, and compare the value of decimals.
- Add, subtract, multiply, and divide decimals.
- Change fractions to decimals and decimals to fractions.

*M*edication dosages and other health care measurements are usually prescribed in the metric measure, which is based on the decimal system. Therefore, it is critical that you understand how to read decimals. A serious medication error can occur if the drug dosage written in a decimal format is misread.

A *decimal* is simply a fraction, written in a different format, with a denominator that is any multiple of

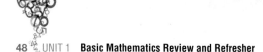

10 (10, 100, and 1,000). The decimal point (.) placement determines the decimal's value. See the following
examples:

EXAMPLES:

Fraction	Decimal	Position to the Right of Decimal	Decimal Point Value
2/10	0.2	1 place	Tenths
3/100	0.03	2 places	Hundredths
4/1,000	0.004	3 places	Thousandths

It is important to remember that numbers to the
right of the decimal point have a value *less than 1*.
Numbers to the left of the decimal point are whole
numbers that have a value equal to or *greater than 1*.
If there is no whole number before the decimal point,
always add a zero (0) to the left of the decimal point
to avoid errors when reading the decimal's value.
Reading decimals is easy once you understand the
concept of decimal values relative to the placement
of the decimal point and whole numbers. Refer to
Figure 3.1 and the following rule.

_R U L E_

Numbers to the right of the decimal point have a *value less
than 1*, and numbers to the left of the decimal point have a
value equal to or greater than 1.

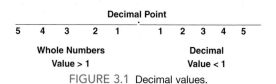

FIGURE 3.1 Decimal values.

RULE

To read decimals: Read the whole number(s) to the left of the decimal point first, read the decimal point as "and" or "point," and then read the decimal fraction to the right of the decimal point. The zero (0) to the left of the decimal point is not read aloud.

EXAMPLES:

0.2 is read as 2 tenths because the number 2 is one position to the right of the decimal point.

0.03 is read as 3 hundredths because the number 3 is two positions to the right of the decimal point.

0.004 is read as 4 thousandths because the number 4 is three positions to the right of the decimal point.

0.150 is read as 15 hundredths because the zero after the 15 does not enhance its value.

EXAMPLES:

Read:

5.2	6.03	0.004
5 . 2	6 . 0 3	0 . 0 0 4

five
and
two tenths

six
and
three hundredths

four thousandths

_R U L E_

To write decimals: Write the whole number (write zero [0]
before the decimal point if there is no whole number), write
the decimal point, and then write the decimal fraction.
Note: Zeros written at the end of the decimal fraction _do
not change_ the decimal's value.

PRACTICE PROBLEMS

*Write the following decimals as you would
read them:*

1. 10.001 _____   2. 3.0007 _____

3. 0.083 _____   4. 0.153 _____

5. 36.0067 _____   6. 0.0125 _____

7. 125.025 _____   8. 20.075 _____

Write the following in decimal format:

9. Five and thirty-seven thousandths

   _____

10. Sixty-four and seven hundredths

   _____

11. Twenty thousandths

   _____

12. Four tenths

   _____

13. Eight and sixty-four thousandths

_____

14. Thirty-three and seven tenths

_____

15. Fifteen thousandths

_____

16. One tenth

_____

Compare Decimal Values

Understanding which decimals are larger or smaller helps prevent serious medication dosage errors. If a patient was prescribed 0.1 mg of a drug, you wouldn't give 0.2 mg.

_R U L E_

To compare decimal values: The decimal with the largest number in the column to the right of the decimal (tenth place) has the greater value. If both are equal, then apply the rule to the next column (hundredth place). This rule also applies to whole numbers.

EXAMPLES:

1. 0.75 is greater than 0.60
2. 0.250 is greater than 0.125
3. 1.36 is greater than 1.25
4. 2.75 is greater than 2.50

PRACTICE PROBLEMS

Select the decimal with the largest value.

1. 0.15   0.25   0.75   _____

2. 0.175   0.186   0.921   _____

3. 1.30   1.35   1.75   _____

4. 2.25   2.40   2.80   _____

Add of Decimals

RULE

To add decimals: Place the decimals in a vertical column with the decimal points directly under one another and add zeros to balance the columns. Start at the far right column. Add the decimals in the same manner as whole numbers are added, and place the decimal in the answer under the aligned decimal points.

EXAMPLE: *Add:* 0.5 + 3.24 + 8

$$\begin{array}{r} 0.50 \\ 3.24 \\ +8.00 \\ \hline \end{array}$$

- Start with the far right column.

- Add the decimals in the same manner as whole numbers are added.

- Place the decimal in the answer directly
  under aligned decimal points.

$$
\begin{array}{r}
0.50 \\
3.24 \\
+8.00 \\
\hline
11.74
\end{array}
$$

ANSWER: 11.74

EXAMPLE: *Add:* 3.9 + 4.7

$$
\begin{array}{r}
3.9 \\
+4.7 \\
\hline
8.6
\end{array}
$$

ANSWER: 8.6

EXAMPLE: *Add:* 6 + 2.8 + 1.6

$$
\begin{array}{r}
6.0 \\
2.8 \\
+1.6 \\
\hline
10.4
\end{array}
$$

ANSWER: 10.4

Subtract of Decimals

RULE

To subtract decimals: Place the decimals in a vertical column with the decimal points directly under one another
and add zeros to balance the columns. Start at the far right
column. Subtract the decimals in the same manner as
whole numbers are subtracted, and place the decimal in
the answer under the aligned decimal points.

EXAMPLE: *Subtract:* 4.1 from 6.2

$$\begin{array}{r} 6.2 \\ -4.1 \end{array}$$

- Start with the far right column.

- Subtract the decimals in the same manner as whole numbers are subtracted. Place the decimal point in the answer directly under the aligned decimal points.

$$\begin{array}{r} 6.2 \\ -4.1 \\ \hline 2.1 \end{array}$$

ANSWER: 2.1

EXAMPLE: *Subtract:* 1.32 from 16.84

$$\begin{array}{r} 16.84 \\ -1.32 \\ \hline 15.52 \end{array}$$

ANSWER: 15.52

EXAMPLE: *Subtract:* 8.00 from 13.60

$$\begin{array}{r} 13.60 \\ -8.00 \\ \hline 5.60 \end{array}$$

ANSWER: 5.60

| EXAMPLE: | *Subtract:* 3.0086 from 7.02 |

$$\begin{array}{r} 7.0200 \\ -\,3.0086 \\ \hline 4.0114 \end{array}$$

ANSWER: 4.0114

Multiply of Decimals

Multiplication of Decimal Numbers

Multiplication of decimals is done using the same method as is used for multiplying whole numbers. The major concern is placement of the decimal point in the product.

___R U L E___

To multiply decimals: Place the decimals in the same position as whole numbers, multiply, and record the product
without decimal points. Count off the number of decimal
places *to the right* of both numbers being multiplied, and
use that number to place the decimal point in the product.
Add zeros on the left if necessary.

| EXAMPLE: | *Multiply:* 6.3 by 7.6 |

$$\begin{array}{r} 6.3 \\ \times\,7.6 \end{array}$$

- Multiply the decimal numbers as you
  would multiply whole numbers. Write
  down the product without the decimal
  point.

$$
\begin{array}{r}
6.3 \\
\times\ 7.6 \\
\hline
378 \\
441 \\
\hline
4788\ \text{(product)}
\end{array}
$$

- Count off the number of decimal places *to the right* of the decimals in the two numbers being multiplied. In this case, there are two places. Count off the total number of places in the product.

$$
\begin{array}{r}
6.3 \\
\times\ 7.6 \\
\hline
378 \\
441 \\
\hline
47.88
\end{array}
$$

6.3   one place to right of decimal

× 7.6   + one place to right of decimal

47.88   two places, counting right to left

Answer: 47.88

Multiplication by 10, 100, or 1,000

Multiplying by 10, 100, or 1,000 is a fast and easy way to calculate dosage problems. Simply move the decimal point the same number of places to the right as there are zeros in the multiplier. See Table 3.1.

EXAMPLE: 0.712×10. There is one zero in the multiplier of 10. Move the decimal one place to the right for an answer of 7.12.

$$0.712 = 0.712 = 7.12$$

Table 3.1 **Multiplying by 10, 100, or 1,000**

Multiplier	Number of Zeros	Move the Decimal to the Right
10	1	1 place
100	2	2 places
1,000	3	3 places

EXAMPLE: $0.08 \times 1,000$. There are three zeros in the multiplier of 1,000. Move the decimal three places to the right for an answer of 80.

$$0.08 = 0.080 = 80$$

Divide of Decimals

Division of Decimal Numbers

To divide decimals, use the same method you would use to divide whole numbers.

When you divide decimals, the most important thing to remember is movement and placement of the decimal point in the divisor (number divided by), dividend (number divided), and quotient (product).

$$\overset{\text{Quotient}}{\text{Divisor}\,)\overline{\text{Dividend}}} \qquad \frac{\text{Dividend}}{\text{Divisor}} = \text{Quotient}$$

$$8\,\overline{)64}^{\,8} \qquad \frac{64}{8} = 8$$

RULE

To divide a decimal by a whole number: Place the decimal point in the quotient directly above the decimal point in the dividend.

EXAMPLE: $25.5 \div 5$

$$
\begin{array}{r}
5.1 \text{ (quotient)} \\
5\overline{)25.5} \\
\underline{25} \\
5 \\
\underline{5}
\end{array}
$$

ANSWER: 5.1

RULE

To divide a decimal by a decimal: Make the decimal number in the divisor a whole number *first,* move the decimal point in the dividend the same number of places that you moved the decimal point in the divisor, place the decimal point in the quotient directly above the decimal point in the dividend, and add a zero in front of the decimal point.

EXAMPLE: To divide 0.32 by 1.6, make 1.6 a whole number (16) by moving the decimal point one place to the right. Move the decimal point in the dividend (0.32) the same number of places (one) that you moved the decimal point in the divisor.

Divide: 3.2 by 16

$$
\begin{array}{r}
.2 \\
16\overline{)3 \uparrow 2} \\
\underline{3.2}
\end{array}
$$

ANSWER: 0.2

Table 3.2 **Dividing by 10, 100, or 1,000**

Divisor	Number of Zeros	Move the Decimal to the Left
10	1	1 place
100	2	2 places
1,000	3	3 places

Division by 10, 100, or 1,000

Dividing by 10, 100, or 1,000 is fast and easy. Just move the decimal point the same number of places *to the left* as there are zeros in the divisor. See Table 3.2.

EXAMPLE: $0.09 \div 10$. Move the decimal one place to the left for an answer of 0.009.

$$0.09 = .009 = 0.009$$

PRACTICE PROBLEMS

Add the following decimals (carry out to hundredths):

1. $16.4 + 21.8 = $ _____

2. $0.009 + 18.4 = $ _____

3. $67.541 + 17.1 = $ _____

4. $0.27 + 1.64 = $ _____

5. $1.01 + 18.9 =$ _____

6. $26.07 + 0.0795 =$ _____

Subtract the following decimals (carry out to hundredths):

7. $366.18 - 122.6 =$ _____

8. $107.16 - 56.1 =$ _____

9. $16.19 - 3.86 =$ _____

10. $15.79 - 9.11 =$ _____

11. $148.22 - 81.97 =$ _____

12. $2.46 - 1.34 =$ _____

Multiply the following decimals (carry out to hundredths):

13. $1.86 \times 12.1 =$ _____

14. $0.89 \times 7.65 =$ _____

15. $13 \times 7.8 =$ _____

16. $10.65 \times 100 =$ _____

17. $19.4 \times 2.16 =$ _____

18. $5.33 \times 1.49 =$ _____

19. $16 \times 9.002 =$ _____

20. $54 \times 7.41 =$ _____

Divide the following decimals (carry out to hundredths):

21. $63.8 \div 0.09 =$ _____

22. $39.7 \div 1.3 =$ _____

23. $98.4 \div 1,000 =$ _____

24. $0.008 \div 10 =$ _____

25. $41 \div 4.4 =$ _____

26. $18.61 \div 7.01 =$ _____

27. $134 \div 12.3 =$ _____

28. $99 \div 7.7 =$ _____

thePoint Additional practice problems to enhance learning and facilitate chapter comprehension can be found at **http://thePoint.lww.com/Boyer8e.**

Change Fractions to Decimals

When changing a fraction to a decimal, the numerator of the fraction (1) is divided by the denominator (5). If a numerator does not divide evenly into the denominator, then work the division to three places.

$$\frac{1}{5} = \frac{\text{numerator}}{\text{denominator}} \quad \text{becomes} \quad \frac{\text{dividend}}{\text{divisor}} = \frac{1}{5} \, 5\overline{)1}$$

___R U L E___

To convert a fraction to a decimal: Rewrite the fraction in division format, place a decimal point after the whole number in the dividend, add zeros, place the decimal point in the quotient directly above the decimal point in the dividend, and divide the number by the denominator. Carry out to three places.

EXAMPLE: Change $\dfrac{1}{5}$ to a decimal.

- Rewrite the fraction in decimal format.

- Place a decimal point after the whole number in the dividend. Add zeros.

- Align decimal point in quotient.

- Divide number by denominator and add zeros, if necessary.

$$\frac{1}{5} = \frac{0.2}{5\overline{)1.0}}$$

ANSWER: 0.2

EXAMPLE: *Convert:* $\dfrac{1}{6} = \dfrac{0.166}{6\overline{)1.000}}$
$$\begin{array}{r} \underline{6} \\ 40 \\ \underline{36} \\ 40 \\ \underline{36} \\ 4 \end{array}$$

ANSWER: 0.166

EXAMPLE:

$$\frac{1}{8} = 1 \div 8 = 8\overline{)1}$$

$$\begin{array}{r} 0.125 \\ 8\overline{)1.000} \\ \underline{8} \\ 20 \\ \underline{16} \\ 40 \\ \underline{40} \\ \end{array}$$

Convert:

ANSWER: 0.125

EXAMPLE:

$$\frac{5}{20} = \frac{1}{4} = 1 \div 4 = 4\overline{)1}$$

$$\begin{array}{r} 0.25 \\ 4\overline{)1.00} \\ \underline{8} \\ 20 \\ \underline{20} \\ \end{array}$$

Convert:

ANSWER: 0.25

Change Decimals to Fractions

RULE

To change a decimal to a fraction: Simply read the decimal and then write it as it sounds. Reduce if necessary.

EXAMPLE: Change 0.75 to a fraction.

Read 0.75 as 75 hundredths

Write as $\dfrac{75}{100}$

Reduce $\dfrac{75}{100}$ to $\dfrac{3}{4}$

EXAMPLE: Change 0.5 to a fraction.

Read 0.5 as 5 tenths

Write as $\dfrac{5}{10}$

Reduce $\dfrac{5}{10}$ to $\dfrac{1}{2}$

Round Off Decimals

Most decimals are "rounded off" to the hundredth place to ensure accuracy of calculations. Because this process is done infrequently in the clinical setting, it is explained in *Appendix B* for those of you who wish to review the steps.

PRACTICE PROBLEMS

Convert the following fractions to decimals:

1. $\dfrac{6}{30}$ _____

2. $\dfrac{8}{64}$ _____

3. $\dfrac{15}{60}$ _____

4. $\dfrac{12}{180}$ _____

5. $\dfrac{16}{240}$ _____

6. $\dfrac{3}{57}$ _____

Convert the following decimals to fractions:

7. 0.007 _____   8. 0.93 _____

9. 0.412 _____   10. 5.03 _____

11. 12.2 _____   12. 0.125 _____

---

thePoint Additional practice problems to enhance
learning and facilitate chapter comprehension can be
found at **http://thePoint.lww.com/Boyer8e.**

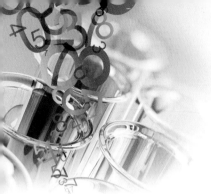

*Write the following decimals as you would
read them:*

1. 5.04 _____   2. 10.65 _____

3. 0.008 _____   4. 18.9 _____

Write the following decimals:

5. Six and eight hundredths

   _____

6. One hundred twenty-four and three tenths

   _____

7. Sixteen and one thousandths

   _____

Solve the following decimal problems:

8. $16.35 + 8.1 =$ _____

9. $0.062 + 59.2 =$ _____

10. $7.006 - 4.23 =$ _____

11. $15.610 - 10.4 =$ _____

12. $27.05 \times 8.3 =$ _____

13. $0.009 \times 14.2 =$ _____

14. $18.75 \div 12 =$ _____

15. $1.070 \div 0.20 =$ _____

16. $12.4 + 3.8 =$ _____

17. $0.893 + 5.88 =$ _____

18. $4.38 - 0.12 =$ _____

19. $12.78 - 4.31 =$ _____

20. $38.02 \times 89.1 =$ _____

21. $12.9 \times 0.06 =$ _____

22. $23.56 \div 0.024 =$ _____

23. $2.109 \div 6.43 =$ _____

Convert the following fractions to decimals and decimals to fractions:

24. $\dfrac{6}{10}$ _____ 25. $\dfrac{12}{84}$ _____

26. $\dfrac{3}{4}$ _____ 27. 0.45 _____

28. 0.75 _____

29. 0.06 _____

30. $\dfrac{8}{20}$ _____

31. $\dfrac{2}{9}$ _____

32. $\dfrac{4}{5}$ _____

33. 6.8 _____

34. 1.35 _____

35. 8.5 _____

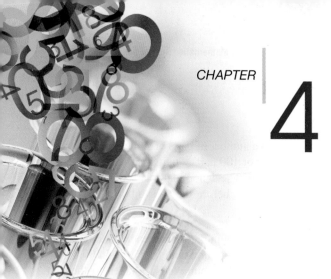

Percents, Ratio, and Proportion

LEARNING OBJECTIVES

After completing this chapter, you should be able to:

- Define the term *percent*.
- Change a percent to a fraction and a fraction to a percent.
- Change a percent to a decimal and a decimal to a percent.
- Determine what percentage one number is of another number.
- Define the terms *ratio* and *proportion*.
- Solve for *x* using ratio and proportion in both the fraction and colon format.

Percent

A *percent*:

- Refers to a number of parts of something, relative to the whole or 100 parts, "parts per hundred."
- Is a fraction. The denominator is 100; the numerator is the number before the % symbol. For example, $5\% = \dfrac{5}{100}$
- Is a ratio. The numerator and denominator are separated by a colon. For example, $5\% = 5{:}100$.
- Is a decimal. The numerator is taken to the hundredth part. For example, $5\% = 0.05$.
- Is written with the symbol %, which means 100.

EXAMPLE: $5\% = \dfrac{5}{100} = 5{:}100 = 0.05$

Percents are commonly used when intravenous solutions are prescribed; e.g., 0.25% and 0.45%. These % solutions refer to the grams of the solute or solid, per 100 parts of solution.

The *percent symbol* can be found with:

- A whole number   20%
- A fraction number   1/2%
- A mixed number   20 1/2%
- A decimal number   20.5%

Fractions and Percents

Sometimes it is necessary to change a percent to a fraction or a fraction to a percent to make dosage calculations easier.

Change a Percent to a Fraction

RULE

To change a percent to a fraction: drop the % symbol, divide the number (new numerator) by 100 (denominator), reduce, and change to a mixed number, if necessary.

EXAMPLE: Change 20% to a fraction

- Drop the % symbol: 20% now becomes 20.

- This number (20) now becomes the fraction's new numerator.

- Place this new numerator (20) over 100 (the denominator will always be 100).

$$20\% = 20 = \frac{20}{100}$$

- Reduce the fraction to lowest terms.

$$\frac{20}{100} = \frac{2}{10} = \frac{1}{5}$$

- Change to a mixed number if necessary.

EXAMPLE: *Change: 40%*

$$40\% = 40 = \frac{40}{100}$$

Reduce: $\quad \frac{40}{100} = \frac{2}{5}$

ANSWER: $\frac{2}{5}$

EXAMPLE: *Change:* $\frac{1}{2}\%$

$$\frac{1}{2}\% = \frac{\frac{1}{2}}{100}$$

$$\frac{1}{2} \div 100 = \frac{1}{2} \times \frac{1}{100} = \frac{1}{200}$$

ANSWER: $\frac{1}{200}$

Change a Fraction to a Percent

RULE

To change a fraction to a percent: multiply the fraction by 100 (change any mixed number to an improper fraction *before* multiplying by 100), reduce, and add the % symbol.

EXAMPLE: *Change:* $\frac{1}{2} = ?$

$$\frac{1}{2} \times \frac{100}{1} = \frac{100}{2} = \frac{50}{1}$$

$$\frac{50}{1} = 50$$

Add % symbol: 50%

> **ANSWER:** 50%

EXAMPLE: *Change:* $\frac{3}{5} = ?$

$$\frac{3}{5} \times 100 = \frac{3}{\cancel{5}_1} \times \cancel{100}^{20}{}_1 = 60$$

Add % symbol: 60%

> **ANSWER:** 60%

EXAMPLE: *Change:* $6\frac{1}{2} = ?$

$$6\frac{1}{2} \times 100$$

Change $6\frac{1}{2}$ to an improper fraction.

$$6\frac{1}{2} = \frac{13}{2}$$

$$\frac{13}{2} \times 100 = \frac{13}{\cancel{2}_1} \times \cancel{100}^{50}{}_1 = 650$$

Add % symbol: 650%

> **ANSWER:** 650%

PRACTICE PROBLEMS

Change the following percents to fractions:

1. 15% _____
2. 30% _____

3. 50% _____
4. 75% _____

5. 25% _____
6. 60% _____

Change the following fractions to percents:

7. $\dfrac{1}{3}$ _____
8. $\dfrac{2}{3}$ _____

9. $\dfrac{1}{5}$ _____
10. $\dfrac{3}{4}$ _____

11. $\dfrac{2}{5}$ _____
12. $\dfrac{1}{4}$ _____

> thePoint₅ Additional practice problems to enhance
> learning and facilitate chapter comprehension can be
> found on **http://thePoint.lww.com/Boyer8e.**

Decimals and Percents

Sometimes it is necessary to change a percent to a
decimal or a decimal to a percent to make dosage
calculations easier.

Change a Percent to a Decimal

_R U L E_

To change a percent to a decimal: drop the % symbol
(when you drop the % symbol from the whole number, a
decimal point takes the place of the symbol), divide the
remaining number by 100 by moving the decimal point _two_
places to the left, and add zeros if necessary.

EXAMPLE:	_Change:_ 68%	Drop the % symbol.
	68% = 68% = 68	Decimal replaces % symbol.
	68.0 = .68. = 0.68	Move the decimal. Add a zero.
		ANSWER: 0.68

EXAMPLE:	_Change:_ 36%	Drop the % symbol.
	36% = 36% = 36	Decimal replaces % symbol.
	36. = .36. = 0.36	Move the decimal. Add a zero.
		ANSWER: 0.36

EXAMPLE:	_Change:_ 14.1%	Drop the % symbol.
	14.1% = 14.1 = 14.1	Decimal replaces % symbol.

$$14.1 = .14.1 = 0.141$$ Move the decimal.

Add a zero.

ANSWER: 0.141

Change a Decimal to a Percent

RULE

To change a decimal to a percent: multiply the decimal by 100 by moving the decimal point two places to the right, and add the % symbol and zeros if needed.

EXAMPLE: *Change:* 3.19

$$3.19 = 3.19. = 319$$ Move the decimal.

Add the % symbol.

ANSWER: 319%

EXAMPLE: *Change:* 1.61

$$1.61 \times 100 = 1.61. = 161$$ Move the decimal.

Add the % symbol.

ANSWER: 161%

EXAMPLE: *Change:* 0.5

$$0.5 \times 100 = 0.50 = 50$$ Move the decimal.

Add the % symbol.

Note: To move the decimal point two places to the right, you need to add a zero.

ANSWER: 50%

Percentage One Number Is of Another Number

RULE

To determine what percentage one number is of another number: make a fraction using the number following "what percent of" as the denominator, use the remaining number as the numerator, change the fraction to a decimal, and then change the decimal to a percent.

EXAMPLE: What percent of 40 is 10?

Convert to a fraction: $\dfrac{10}{40}$

Change to a decimal: $\dfrac{10}{40} = \dfrac{1}{4} = 0.25$

Change to a percent: $0.25 = 25\%$

EXAMPLE: What percent of 60 is 20?

Convert to a fraction: $\dfrac{20}{60}$

Change to a decimal: $\dfrac{20}{60} = \dfrac{2}{6} = \dfrac{1}{3} = 0.33$

Change to a percent: $0.33 = 33\%$

PRACTICE PROBLEMS

Change the following percents to decimals:

1. 15% _____   2. 25% _____

3. 59% _____   4. 80% _____

Change the following decimals to percents:

5. 0.25 _____   6. 0.45 _____

7. 0.60 _____   8. 0.85 _____

Determine the percentage one number is of another number.

9. What percent of 90 is 15? _____

10. What percent of 4 is 1/2? _____

11. What percent of 25 is 5? _____

12. What percent of 180 is 60? _____

> thePoint, Additional practice problems to enhance learning and facilitate chapter comprehension can be found on **http://thePoint.lww.com/Boyer8e.**

Ratio and Proportion

A ratio is the same as a fraction: it indicates division. A ratio is used to express a relationship between one unit or part of the whole. A slash (/) or colon (:) is used to indicate division, and both are read as "is to" or "per."

The *numerator (N) of the fraction is always to the left* of the colon or slash, and the *denominator (D) of the fraction is always to the right* of the colon or slash.

With medications, a ratio usually refers to the weight of a drug (e.g., grams) in a solution (e.g., mL). Therefore, 50 mg/mL = 50 mg of a drug (solute) in 1 mL of a liquid (solution). For the ratio of 1 part to a total of 2 parts, you can write 1:2 or 1/2.

EXAMPLES: $1:2 = 1/2 = \dfrac{1}{2}$

$2:5 = 2/5 = \dfrac{2}{5}$

$3:6 = 3/6 = \dfrac{3}{6} = \dfrac{1}{2}$

A Proportion Expressed as a Fraction

A *proportion* is two ratios that are equal. A proportion can be written in the fraction or colon format. In the *fraction format*, the numerator and the denominator of one fraction have the same relationship as the numerator and denominator of another fraction (they are equivalent). The equals symbol (=) is read as "as" or "equals."

EXAMPLE: $\left.\dfrac{1}{3} = \dfrac{3}{9}\right\}$ 1 is to 3 as 3 is to 9

A Proportion Expressed in the Colon Format

In the *colon format*, the ratio to the left of the double colon is equal to the ratio to the right of the double colon. The double colon (::) is read as "as." You can also use an equals symbol (=). The first and fourth terms are called *extremes* and the second and third terms are called the *means*.

EXTREMES

$$\overbrace{1:3 :: 3:9}$$

MEANS

EXAMPLE: 1:3 :: 3:9}   1 is to 3 as 3 is to 9

1:3 = 3:9}   1 is to 3 equals 3 is to 9

_R U L E_

To verify that two ratios are equal: multiply the means and then multiply the extremes. The product of the means must always equal the product of the extremes.

EXAMPLE: 1:3 :: 3:9

$$\overbrace{1:3 :: 3:9}$$

$1 \times 9 = 9$

$3 \times 3 = 9$

$9 = 9$

ANSWER: 9

_R U L E_

To verify that two fractions are equal: cross-multiply the numerator of each fraction by its opposite denominator and the products will be equal.

EXAMPLE:

$$\frac{1}{3} : \frac{3}{9}$$

$$\frac{1}{3} \diagdown \diagup \frac{3}{9}$$

$$1 \times 9 = 9$$

$$3 \times 3 = 9$$

$$9 = 9$$

ANSWER: 9

Use of Ratio and Proportion: Solving for *x*

To review, a *ratio* expresses the relationship of one unit/quantity to another. A *proportion* expresses the relationship between two ratios that are equal. Sometimes you will have to solve a proportion problem with one unknown quantity, known as *x*. If the proportion is written in the colon format, multiply the means and then the extremes. Try to keep the unknown *x* on the left. If the proportion is written in the fraction format, you need to cross-multiply and then divide to solve for *x*.

Solving for *x* Using a Fraction Format

RULE

To solve for *x*: cross-multiply the numerator of each fraction by its opposite denominator, remembering to *keep the x on the left*. Divide both sides of the equation by the number before the *x*.

EXAMPLE: $\dfrac{1}{3} = \dfrac{x}{9}$ $x = $ unknown

Cross-multiply: $3 \times x = 9 \times 1$

$3x = 9$

Divide both sides of the equation by the number before the x (3).

Divide: $\dfrac{{}^{1}\cancel{3}x}{\cancel{3}_1} = \dfrac{\cancel{9}^{3}}{\cancel{3}_1}$

Reduce: $x = \dfrac{3}{1}$

$x = 3$

ANSWER: 3

EXAMPLES: $\dfrac{2}{5} = \dfrac{x}{20}$ $5x = 40$ $x = 8$

$\dfrac{1/2}{10} = \dfrac{x}{40}$ $10x = 20$ $x = 2$

$\dfrac{36}{12} = \dfrac{x}{2}$ $12x = 72$ $x = 6$

Note: Because the number *before* the x is the same in the numerator and denominator of one ratio, these numbers will cross themselves out and equal 1. Therefore, a shortcut is to *move the number before the x to the denominator on the opposite side.* This quick process is especially important when solving for x in dosage calculation problems.

Solving for x Using a Colon Format

___RULE___

To solve for *x:* write what you have or know in the colon format (25 : 5), and then write what you desire or the unknown in colon format (50 : *x*). Therefore, 25 : 5 = 50 : *x*. Multiply the extremes (25 × *x*), which keeps the *x* on the left, and then multiply the means (5 × 50). Then solve for *x*.

A medication example will be presented next in order to illustrate how to apply the concept of *solving for x*, using ratio and proportion, for drug dosage problems.

Applying the Concept of Solving for x Using a Sample Dosage Problem

Frequently in dosage calculation problems, one quantity is known (100 mg/mL), and it is necessary to find an unknown quantity because the physician has ordered something different from what is available (75 mg). The unknown quantity (? mL necessary to give 75 mg) is identified as *x*.

The following medication problem will be solved using both the fraction and decimal/colon format.

EXAMPLE: Demerol, 75 mg, is prescribed for postoperative pain. The medication is available as 100 mg/mL. To administer the prescribed dose of 75 mg, the nurse would give _____ mL.

- For the fraction format, always write down what is available or *what you have.* You are expressing the ratio relationship of one quantity (mg) to another quantity (mL). *Remember,* the unit of measurement in the numerator of the fraction must be the same for both fractions. The unit of measurement in the denominator of the fraction also must be the same for both fractions.

$$\frac{100 \text{ mg}}{1 \text{ mL}}$$

- Complete the proportion by writing down what you desire (what the physician had ordered), making sure that the numerators are like units and the denominators are like units in the fraction ratios used.

$$\frac{\text{mg}}{\text{mL}} :: \frac{\text{mg}}{\text{mL}} = \frac{100 \text{ mg}}{1 \text{ mL}} :: \frac{75 \text{ mg}}{x \text{ mL}}$$

- Cross-multiply the numerator of each fraction by its opposite denominator and *drop the terms used for units of measurement.*

$$\frac{100 \text{ mg}}{1 \text{ mL}} \diagdown\kern-0.8em\diagup \frac{75 \text{ mg}}{x \text{ mL}}$$

- Complete the proportion:

$$100 \times x = 75 \times 1$$
$$100x = 75$$

- Solve for *x* by dividing both sides of the equation by the number before *x*. In this case, the number before *x* is 100, so divide both sides of the equation by 100. Convert your answer to a decimal, which is easier to work with than a fraction. Refer to the beginning of this chapter to review the traditional and abbreviated methods for solving for *x*. For the purpose of brevity, an abbreviated method will be used throughout the remainder of the book.

$$\frac{^1\cancel{100}x}{_1\cancel{100}} = \frac{75}{100}$$

$$x = \frac{75}{100}$$

- Reduce: $\dfrac{75}{100} = \dfrac{3}{4}$ mL or 0.75 mL

ANSWER: 3/4 or 0.75 mL

EXAMPLE: Demerol in 75 mg is prescribed for post-operative pain. The medication is available as 100 mg/mL. To administer the prescribed dose of 75 mg, the nurse would have to give _____ mL.

- For the decimal/colon format, always write down what is available or *what you have. Remember,* the unit of measurement to the left of the colon must be the same for both ratios; the unit of measurement to the right of the colon must be the same for both ratios. For this example, you should write:

100 mg : 1 mL

- Complete the proportion by writing down *what you desire*, making sure that both ratios are written in the same format.

$$100 \text{ mg} : 1 \text{ mL} = 75 \text{ mg} : x \text{ mL}$$

- Multiply the extremes:

$$\overline{ \text{EXTREMES} }$$

$$100 \text{ mg} : 1 \text{ mL} :: 75 \text{ mg} : x \text{ mL}$$

$$(100 \text{ mg} \times x \text{ mL} =)$$

- Multiply the means:

$$100 \text{ mg} : 1 \text{ mL} :: 75 \text{ mg} : x \text{ mL}$$

$$\underline{\text{MEANS}\underline{}}$$

$$(= 75 \text{ mg} \times 1 \text{ mL})$$

- Complete the equation ($100 \text{ mg} \times x \text{ mL} = 75 \text{ mg} \times 1 \text{ mL}$) and *drop the units of measurement.*

$$100x = 75$$

- Solve for x. (Remember: divide both sides of the equation by the number before x [100].) Convert your answer to a decimal.

$$\frac{100x}{100} = \frac{75}{100}$$

$$\frac{\overset{1}{\cancel{100}}x}{\underset{1}{\cancel{100}}} = \frac{75}{100}$$

$$x = \frac{75}{100}$$

- Reduce: $\dfrac{75}{100} = \dfrac{3}{4}$ mL or 0.75 mL

ANSWER: 3/4 or 0.75 mL

Verify Accuracy

RULE

To verify the accuracy of an answer obtained by solving for *x*, determine that the sum products are equal.

Verify the accuracy of the answer, $x = 0.75$ mL.

- For the *fraction format,* multiply the numerator of each ratio by its opposite denominator. The sum products will be equal.

$$\dfrac{100 \text{ mg}}{1 \text{ mL}} :: \dfrac{75 \text{ mg}}{\dfrac{3}{4} \text{ mL}}$$

$$\left.\begin{array}{l} {}^{25}\cancel{100} \times \dfrac{3}{\cancel{4}_1} = 75 \\[2mm] 1 \times 75 = 75 \end{array}\right\} \begin{array}{l} \text{Sum products} \\ \text{are equal} \end{array}$$

- For the *colon format,* multiply the extremes and then multiply the means. The product of the means will equal the product of the extremes.

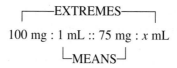

$$\text{EXTREMES}$$
$$100 \text{ mg} : 1 \text{ mL} :: 75 \text{ mg} : x \text{ mL}$$
$$\text{MEANS}$$

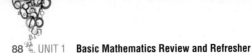
$$75 \times 1 \text{ mL} = 75$$

$$100 \times \frac{3}{4} = \frac{\overset{25}{\cancel{100}}}{1} \times \frac{3}{\underset{1}{\cancel{4}}} = 75 \qquad \left.\begin{array}{l} \text{Sum products} \\ \text{are equal} \end{array}\right\}$$

Critical Thinking Check

If 75 mg is prescribed and 100 mg/mL is available, does it seem logical that the quantity to be given would be less than 1.0 mL? _____ **Yes or No?**

PRACTICE PROBLEMS

Write the following relationships in ratio format, using both the fraction and colon format:

1. Pediatric drops contain 50 mg/5 mL.

2. There are 325 mg in each tablet.

3. A liter of IV solution contains 2 ampules of multivitamins.

4. A capsule contains 250 mg of a drug.

Write the following relationships as proportions, using both the fraction and colon format:

5. Each tablet contains 5 grains of a drug. The nurse is to give 3 tablets equal to 15 grains.

6. A drug is available in 0.2-mg tablets. A patient is prescribed 0.4 mg/day provided by 2 tablets.

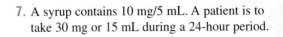

7. A syrup contains 10 mg/5 mL. A patient is to take 30 mg or 15 mL during a 24-hour period.

Use ratio and proportion to solve for x.

8. $\dfrac{4}{12} = \dfrac{3}{x}$ _____

9. $\dfrac{6}{x} = \dfrac{9}{27}$ _____

10. $\dfrac{2}{7} = \dfrac{x}{14}$ _____

11. $\dfrac{5}{25} = \dfrac{10}{x}$ _____

12. If 50 mg of a drug is available in 1 mL of solution, how many milliliters would contain 40 mg?

    Set up ratio: proportion and solve for *x:* _____

13. A drug is available as 25 mg/mL.

    To give 1.5 mL, you would give _____ mg.

    Set up ratio: proportion and solve for *x:* _____

14. A tablet contains 0.125 mg.

    The nurse gave 2 tablets or _____ mg.

    Set up ratio: proportion and solve for *x:* _____

15. An oral liquid is available as 1 gram in each 5 mL.

    The nurse gave 15 mL or _____ grams.

    Set up ratio: proportion and solve for *x:* _____

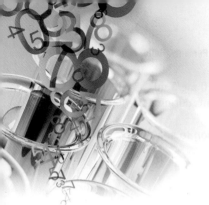

Change the following:

	Percent	Fraction	Decimal
1.	_____	1/6	_____
2.	_____	_____	0.25
3.	6.4%	_____	_____
4.	21%	_____	_____
5.	_____	2/5	_____
6.	_____	_____	1.62
7.	_____	_____	0.27
8.	5 1/4%	_____	_____
9.	_____	9/2	_____
10.	8 3/9%	_____	_____
11.	1%	_____	_____
12.	_____	6/7	_____

13. _____   18/4   _____

14. _____   _____   1.5

15. _____   _____   0.72

Write the following ratios in fraction and colon format:

16. A tablet contains 10 mg of a drug.

_____ fraction _____ colon

17. A liquid is available for injection as 10 units in each milliliter.

_____ fraction _____ colon

18. A physician ordered 200 mg of a drug per kilogram of body weight.

_____ fraction _____ colon

19. The physician ordered 300 mg of a drug, which was available in 100-mg tablets.

_____ fraction _____ colon

20. A physician ordered 500 mg of a drug. The medication was available in 250-mg tablets.

_____ fraction _____ colon

21. A drug is available in 0.075-mg tablets. A physician ordered 0.15 mg daily.

_____ fraction _____ colon

22. A physician ordered 500 mg of a liquid medication that was available as 250 mg/0.5 mL.

_____ fraction _____ colon

Solve for x, using ratios and proportions.

23. If $\dfrac{1}{50} = \dfrac{x}{40}$ then $x =$

24. If $\dfrac{6}{18} = \dfrac{2}{x}$ then $x =$

25. If $\dfrac{x}{12} = \dfrac{9}{24}$ then $x =$

26. If $\dfrac{3}{9} = \dfrac{x}{18}$ then $x =$

Solve for x for the remaining problems and verify your answers using a fraction or colon format: use a critical thinking check to evaluate the logic of your answer.

27. The physician prescribed 10 mg of a day. The medication was available as 20 mg/mL. The nurse would give _____ mL.

    Verify your answer: _____

C r i t i c a l   T h i n k i n g   C h e c k

If one-half the available dosage is prescribed, then does it seem logical that the quantity to be given would be less than 1.0 mL? _____ **Yes or No?**

28. The physician prescribed 25 mg of a syrup to be
    given every 3 hours for pain as needed. The syrup
    was available as 50 mg/5 mL. To give 25 mg, the
    nurse would give _____ mL.

    Verify your answer: _____

Critical Thinking Check

If one-half the available dosage (50 mg/5 mL) is
prescribed, then does it seem logical that the
quantity to be given would be less than 3 mL?
_____ **Yes or No?**

29. The physician ordered 1.5 mg of an injectable liq-
    uid. The medication was available as 3.0 mg/mL.
    The nurse would give _____ mL.

    Verify your answer: _____

Critical Thinking Check

If one-half the available dosage is prescribed
(3 mg/1 mL), then does it seem logical that the
quantity to be given would be less than 1 mL?
_____ **Yes or No?**

30. The physician prescribed 25 mg of a one-dose
    injectable liquid. The drug was available as 20 mg/
    2 mL. The nurse would give _____ mL.

    Verify your answer: _____

Critical Thinking Check

If an additional 25% of the available dosage (20 mg/2 mL) is prescribed, does it seem logical that the quantity to be given would be greater than 3 mL? _____ **Yes or No?**

31. The physician prescribed 30 mg of an oral solution available as 20 mg/5 mL. The nurse would give _____ mL.

32. The physician prescribed 40 mg of a solution that was available as 80 mg/15 mL. To give 40 mg, the nurse would give _____ mL.

33. The physician prescribed 7.5 mg of a medication that was available as 15 mg/mL. The nurse would give _____ mL.

34. The physician prescribed 0.6 mg of a medication that was available as 0.4 mg/mL. To give 0.6 mg, the nurse would give _____ mL.

35. The physician prescribed 80 mg of a medication that was available as 100 mg/2 mL. The nurse would give _____ mL.

36. The physician ordered 35 mg of a liquid that was available as 50 mg/mL. The nurse would give _____ mL.

37. The physician ordered 60 mg of a drug that was available as 20 mg/tablet. The nurse would give _____ tablets.

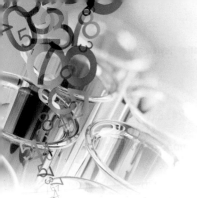

Solve the following problems and reduce each answer to its lowest terms.

1. 1/4 + 3/4 _____
2. 2/3 − 3/5 _____

3. 1/10 + 3/5 _____
4. 3/4 − 1/3 _____

5. 2/6 × 4/5 _____
6. 3/8 × 1/6 _____

7. 1/50 × 20/30 _____
8. 1/100 × 20/30 _____

9. 1/3 ÷ 1/6 _____
10. 1/10 ÷ 1/8 _____

11. 1/12 ÷ 1/3 _____
12. 1/15 ÷ 3/150 _____

Choose the fraction with the highest value in each of the following.

13. 1/3 or 1/4 _____
14. 1/8 or 1/6 _____

15. 1/100 or 1/200 _____
16. 3/30 or 5/30 _____

Solve the following and carry to the nearest hundredths.

17. 1.5 + 1.6 _____
18. 0.46 + 3.8 _____

19. 0.6 − 0.2 _____
20. 6 − 0.32 _____

21. 0.25 × 10_____   22. 0.15 × 100 _____

23. 7.5 ÷ 0.45_____   24. 8.5 ÷ 4.5 _____

Change the following fractions to decimals and decimals to fractions.

25. 8/10 _____   26. 5/20 _____

27. 3/9 _____   28. 0.5 _____

29. 0.07 _____   30. 1.5 _____

Change the following percents to fractions and fractions to percents.

31. 25% _____   32. 1/3% _____

33. 0.6% _____   34. 2/5 _____

35. 4 1/2 _____   36. 1/50 _____

Solve for the value of x in each ratio and proportion problem. Reduce all fractions to their lowest terms or carry all decimals to the hundredths or tenths. Verify your answers.

37. $3 : x = 4 : 16$ _____

38. $25 : 1.5 = 20 : x$ _____

39. $8 : 1 = 10 : x$ _____

40. $4/5 : 25 = x : 50$ _____

41. $0.25 : 500 = x : 1,000$ _____

42. $x : 20 = 2.5 : 100$ _____

43. $10 : 30 = 60 : x$ _____

44. $1/2 : 8 = 1/8 : x$ _____

45. $3 : x = 9 : 1/3$ _____

46. $125 : 250 = 300 : x$ _____

47. $1/2 : x = 1/4 : 0.8$ _____

48. $1/5 : 10 = 1/10 : x$ _____

49. $1/100 : 5 = 1/150 : x$ _____

50. $15 : x = 25 : 150$ _____

51. $8 : x = 48 : 6$ _____

52. $4 : 8 = x : 0.5$ _____

53. $1.5 : 2 = x : 2.5$ _____

54. $20 : x = 80 : 8$ _____

55. $1/75 : 1/150 = 2 : x$ _____

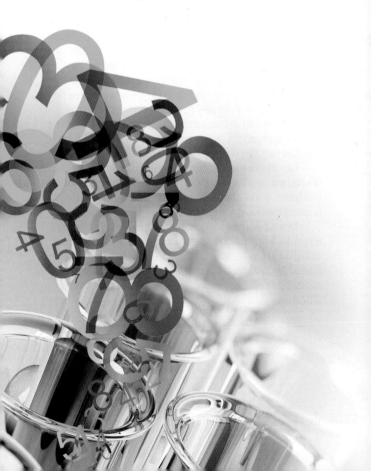

Measurement | 2
Systems

*T*here are three systems of measurement in use today: the metric, household, and apothecary systems. The metric system is the recommended system of choice for dosage calculations because it is the most accurate and consistent. The household system, which is used most frequently in home settings, is inaccurate because of the variations in household measuring devices. The apothecary system is being phased out because it is an approximate system that is not as exact as the metric system and its use of symbols and Roman numerals is confusing. The Joint Commission on the Accreditation of Healthcare Organizations (JCAHO) and the Institute for Safe Medication Practices (ISMP) have both recommended that the apothecary system not be used. (You can read more about safe medication delivery at http://www.ismp.org.) However, because the apothecary system is still used by physicians (drugs ordered in grains and minims) and two common measurement items (medicine cups and syringes) still include apothecary units, this system will be presented here along with the metric and household systems.

Each measurement system has three basic measures: weight, volume, and length. Drugs are commonly prescribed by weight (milligrams, grams, grains) and volume (milliliters, ounces). Length is usually used for assessment (inches, millimeters, and centimeters).

To effectively deliver medications, nurses need to be familiar with all three systems of measurement and become experts at converting one unit of measure to another within the same system or between two systems. In this unit you will be shown how to convert all measurements. Equivalent values have been listed to facilitate conversions and dosage calculations.

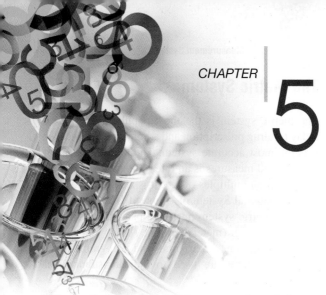

The Metric, Household, and Apothecary Systems of Measurement

LEARNING OBJECTIVES

After completing this chapter, you should be able to:

- List the common rules for metric, household, and apothecary notations.
- Distinguish between the three basic units of measure: length (meter), weight (gram), and volume (liter) for each system.
- Make conversions within each system.

The Metric System

The metric system is the most popular system used today for drug prescription and administration because it is the most accurate system. The metric system of weights and measures is an international decimal system based on multiples of ten. It is also referred to as the International System of Units (SI Units).

The metric system has three basic units of measurement: length (meter), volume (liter), and weight (gram, milligram, microgram and kilogram). Five common prefixes are used to indicate subunits of measure:

> micro = one millionth = mcg
> milli = one thousandth = m
> centi = one hundredth = c
> deci = one tenth = deci
> kilo = one thousand = kg

In the metric system, portions can be increased (multiplied) or decreased (divided) by multiples of 10 (10, 100, 1,000). Conversions are achieved by moving the decimal point to the right for multiplication or to the left for division. For example:

1.0 *increased by* 10 = 1.0 = 10

100 *increased by* 10 = 100.0 = 1,000

0.1 *decreased by* 10 = 0.1 = 0.01

100 *decreased by* 10 = 100. = 10

Common Rules for Metric Notations

RULE

Metric abbreviations always follow the unit amount or numbers.

    0.2 mL   10 kg

RULE

Metric abbreviations are written in lowercase letters except for the abbreviation for *liter,* for which the "L" is capitalized.

    g = gram
    mL = milliliter

RULE

Fractional units are expressed as decimals.

    0.5 mL *not* 1/2 mL

RULE

Zeros are used *in front of* the decimal point when not preceded by a whole number to emphasize the decimal. Omit unnecessary zeros so the dosage is not misread.

    0.5 mL *not* 0.50 mL
    1 mL *not* 1.0 mL

Meter—Length

The meter is:

- The basic unit of *length*
- Equal to 39.37 inches
- Abbreviated as m

The primary linear measurements used in medicine are centimeters (cm) and millimeters (mm). Square meters are used for body surface area (m^2). Centimeters are used for calculating body surface area and measuring such things as the size of body organs, tumors, and wounds. Millimeters are used for blood pressure measurements.

Liter—Volume

The liter is:

- The basic unit of *volume*
- The total volume of liquid in a cube that measures 10 cm $\times$ 10 cm $\times$ 10 cm (1,000 = cm^3)
- Equal to 1,000 mL
- Has a mass (1 L of water) equal to one kilogram (1 kg) at 4°C (degrees Celsius)
- Abbreviated as L

Gram—Weight

The gram is:

- The basic unit of *weight*
- The most widely used unit of measurement for food products

Table 5.1   **Common Metric Measurements and Equivalents**

1 gram (g)	=	1,000 milligrams (mg)
1 milligram (mg)	=	1,000 micrograms (mcg)
1 kilogram (kg)	=	1,000 grams (g)
1 liter (L)	=	1,000 milliliters (mL)
1 meter (m)	=	$\begin{cases} 100 \text{ centimeters (cm)} \\ 1,000 \text{ millimeters (mm)} \end{cases}$

- One, one-thousandths of the SI base unit of a kilogram
- Equal to a volume of 1 mL
- Abbreviated as g

Refer to Table 5.1 for common metric measures and equivalents.

The Apothecary System

Once the first system of measurement for medications, the apothecary system is *not recommended* for use today. The use of symbols and fractions is confusing and can lead to errors. Sometimes a medication label indicates grains, and the metric equivalent is in milligrams. Because the apothecary system may still be used in some instances, it is presented here.

The apothecary system uses approximate measures, fractions (for amounts less than 1), Arabic numbers, and Roman numerals (see Appendix A). The abbreviation "gr" is used for grain, the only unit of weight in this system. The symbols for the liquid measures of dram and ounce are no longer used; this is to avoid medication errors. If medications are ordered in drams or ounces, the words "drams" and "ounces" are written out. The abbreviation "gtt" is used for drop (see Chapter 10) and "m" for minim, which can be found on some syringes. One-half can be abbreviated ss or s̄s̄.

It is helpful to understand the relationship of these terms to the concepts of weight and volume. The original standard measurement of a grain was an amount equal to the weight of a grain of wheat. The minim is considered equal to the quantity of water in a drop that also weighs 1 grain. A dram is equal to 4 mL; an ounce is equal to 30 mL.

Common Rules for the Apothecary System

RULE

Lowercase Roman numerals are used to express whole numbers.

　　3 = iii　　　6 = vi

RULE

Arabic numbers are used for larger quantities (except for 5, 10, and 20) or when the amount is written out.

　　12 ounces

RULE

The apothecary abbreviation/word *always goes before* the quantity.

　　gr x = 10 grains
　　drams viii = 8 drams

_R U L E_

Fractions are used to express quantities that are less than 1 (e.g., gr 1/3). The abbreviation ss or $\overline{ss}$ may be encountered for the fraction 1/2; however, its use is not recommended.

Refer to Table 5.2 for apothecary units of weight and volume.

Household Measurements

Household measurements are calculated by using containers easily found in the home. Common household measuring devices are those utensils used for cooking, eating, and measuring liquid proportions. They include medicine droppers, teaspoons, tablespoons, cups, and glasses. Because containers in the home differ in design, size, and capacity, it is impossible to establish a standard unit of measure. Patients should always be

Table 5.2   **Common Apothecary Units of Weight and Volume**

Unit	Weight or Volume	Abbreviation or Term
Grain		gr
Drop	One drop of water	gtt
Minim	One drop	m
Dram	60 grains	dram
Ounce	8 drams or 30 mL	ounce
Pound	12 ounces*	lb

*In this system a pound is slightly less (12 ounces) than the 16 ounces in the household system.

Table 5.3   **Common Household Quantities and
             Metric Equivalents**

Unit	Volume	Abbreviation	Metric Equivalent
Drop	—	gtt	—
Teaspoon	60 drops	tsp	5 mL
Tablespoon	3 tsp	tbsp	15 mL
Ounce	2 tbsp	oz	30 mL
Tea cup	6 ounces	c	180 mL
Measuring cup	8 ounces	C	240 mL
Pint	16 ounces	pt	500 mL
Quart	2 pt	qt	1,000 mL
Gallon	4 qt	gal	

advised to first use measuring cups or droppers packaged with medications.

It is expected that the household measurement system will increase as health care continues to move into the home and community. The nurse or health care provider will have to teach the patient and family how to measure the amount of medication prescribed, so every effort needs to be made to be as exact as possible. Refer to Table 5.3.

Probably the *most common* measuring device found in the home is the measuring cup, which calibrates ounces and is available for liquid and dry measures (Figure 5.1). Some pharmaceutical companies package 1-ounce measuring cups or calibrated medicine droppers with their over-the-counter medications (e.g., NyQuil, Children's Tylenol). A medication dropper (sometimes supplied with the prescription) marked in mg and mL or an oral syringe marked in teaspoons is commonly used for children (Figure 5.2).

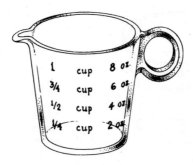

FIGURE 5.1 Standard liquid measuring cup (8–ounce capacity)—a common household container.

Common Rule for the Household System

RULE

Arabic whole numbers and fractions *precede* the unit of measure.

> ¼ cup   8 ounces   3 cups   2 pints

The household system of measurement uses Arabic whole numbers and fractions to precede the unit of measure. Standard cookbook abbreviations are also used (tsp, tbsp, oz). The basic unit of this system is the drop (gtt). A drop is equal to a drop, regardless of the liquid's viscosity (sticky or gummy consistency).

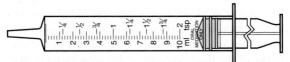

FIGURE 5.2 Oral dosage syringe. (From Craig, G. [2009]. *Clinical Calculations Made Easy* [4th ed.]. Philadelphia: Lippincott Williams & Wilkins.)

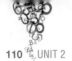

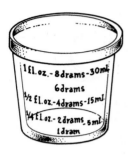

1 fl.oz. - 8 drams - 30 ml
6 drams
½ fl.oz. - 4 drams - 15 ml
¼ fl.oz. - 2 drams 5 ml
1 dram

FIGURE 5.3 One-ounce medicine cup commonly used in hospitals. Indicates household, apothecary, and metric equivalents.

Therefore, when medicine needs to be given in drops, a standard dropper should be used. Household measurements are approximate in comparison to the exactness of the metric and apothecary systems. Hospitals use a standard 1-ounce medicine cup (Figure 5.3). These calibrated containers provide metric, apothecary, and household system equivalents.

RULE

When measuring a liquid medication in a household container, determine the container's capacity *prior to preparing* the medication.

When measuring a liquid medication, it is important that the container/dropper be held so that the calibrations are at eye level. When a container/dropper is held at eye level, the liquid will appear to be uneven or U-shaped. This curve, called a *meniscus,* is caused by surface tension; its shape is influenced by the viscosity of the fluid. Read the calibration at the bottom of the meniscus when measuring the level of a liquid medication. See Figure 5.4.

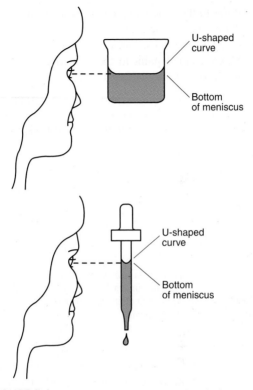

FIGURE 5.4 Liquid medication being read at the bottom of the meniscus; the container or dropper is held at eye level.

Converting Within the Same System: Metric System

Converting or changing units in the metric system is easily done by moving the decimal point. If you choose, you can always use ratio and proportion.

Refer to the following diagram to understand the concept of moving the decimal point when converting dosages. The liter is used as an example.

Move decimal point to the right (larger unit to smaller unit): multiply numeral by 10:

1	10	100	1000

———————————————————————→

1 liter = 10 deciliters = 100 centiliters = 1,000 milliliters

Move decimal point to the left (smaller unit to larger unit): divide numeral by 10:

1	10	100	1000

←———————————————————————

1 liter = 10 deciliters = 100 centiliters = 1,000 milliliters

R U L E

To move *from a smaller* unit *to a larger* unit within the same system: *Divide* the numeral by moving the decimal point *to the left* the number of places to be moved (move one place for each increment).

EXAMPLE: Change millimeters (6,000) to decimeters. To move from milli to deci, you need to move the decimal point two places *to the left.*

60.00 = 60

(milli) = (deci)

ANSWER: 60 dm

RULE

To move *from a larger* unit *to a smaller* unit within the same system: *Multiply* the numeral by moving the decimal point *to the right* the number of places to be moved (move one place for each increment of 10).

EXAMPLE: Change decimeters (80) to centimeters. To move from deci to centi, you need to move the decimal point one place *to the right*.

80.0. = 800
   └↑

(deci) = (centi)

ANSWER: 800 cm

PRACTICE PROBLEMS

Change the following units of metric length, volume, and weight:

1. 3.60 cm = _____ m

2. 4.16 m = _____ dm

3. 0.8 mm = _____ cm

4. 2 mm = _____ m

5. 20.5 mm = _____ cm

6. 18 cm = _____ mm

7. 30 dm = _____ mm

8. 2 cm = _____ m

9. 6 cm = _____ mm

10. 10 dm = _____ m

11. 3.6 mL = _____ L

12. 6.17 cL = _____ mL

13. 0.9 L = _____ mL

14. 6.40 cg = _____ mg

15. 1,000 mg = _____ g

16. 0.8 mg = _____ dg

17. 8 g = _____ cg

18. 16 dL = _____ mL

19. 41.6 mL = _____ L

20. 32 dg = _____ mg

Converting Within the Same System: Household and Apothecary

Conversions within the same system for the apothecary system and household measures *require the memorization of common equivalents,* which can be found in Tables 5.2 and 5.3. There is a standard rule to use to convert units *within the same system,* using ratio and proportion. Converting *between systems* will be covered in Chapter 6.

R U L E

To change units within the same system: Determine equivalent values, write down in a fraction or colon format *what you know* followed by *what you desire,* and solve for *x.*

EXAMPLE #1:

- Select the equivalent values in the system. If you want to know how many milliliters (mL) there are in 2.5 ounces, look up the equivalent value of 30 mL = 1 ounce (Table 5.3).

- Write down *what you know* in a colon or fraction format:

$$\frac{30 \text{ mL}}{1 \text{ ounce}} \quad \text{or} \quad 30 \text{ mL} : 1 \text{ ounce}$$

- Write down *what you desire* in a colon or fraction format to complete the proportion. The numerators and denominators must be the same units of measurement. The answer x will be in ounces.

$$\frac{30 \text{ mL}}{1 \text{ ounce}} :: \frac{x \text{ mL}}{2.5 \text{ ounces}}$$

or

$$30 \text{ mL} : 1 \text{ ounce} = x \text{ mL} : 2.5 \text{ ounces}$$

- Cross-multiply (fraction format) or multiply the extremes and then the means (colon format). Remember: The unit used for an answer will be mL.

$$30 \text{ mL} : 1 \text{ ounce} = x \text{ mL} : 2.5 \text{ ounces}$$
$$x \text{ mL} = 30 \times 2.5$$
$$x \text{ mL} = 75 \text{ mL}$$

EXAMPLE #2: Select the equivalent values in the system (see Table 5.3). If you want to know how many ounces there are in 4 tablespoons, look up the equivalent value of 1 ounce = 2 tablespoons.

- Write down *what you know* in a fraction or colon format.

$$\frac{2 \text{ tbs}}{1 \text{ oz}} \quad \text{or} \quad 2 \text{ tbs} : 1 \text{ oz}$$

- Write down *what you desire* in a fraction or colon format to complete the proportion. The answer x will be in ounces. The numerators and denominators must be the same units of measurement.

$$\frac{2 \text{ tbs}}{1 \text{ oz}} :: \frac{4 \text{ tbs}}{x \text{ oz}}$$

or

$$2 \text{ tbs} : 1 \text{ oz} = 4 \text{ tbs} : x \text{ oz}$$

- Cross-multiply (fraction format) or multiply the extremes and then the means (colon format). Remember: The unit used for an answer will be in ounces.

$$2 \text{ tbs} \times 1 \text{ ounce} = 4 \text{ tbs} \times x \text{ ounces}$$
$$2x = 4$$

- Solve for x:

$$\frac{2x}{2} = \frac{4}{2}$$

$$\frac{2^1 x}{2_1} = \frac{4}{2}$$

$$x = \frac{4^2}{2_1} = 2$$

ANSWER: 2 ounces

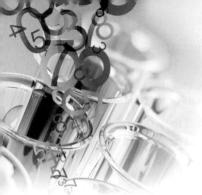

Change the following units of metric length:

1. 7.43 mm = _____ m   2. 0.06 cm = _____ dm

3. 10 km = _____ m   4. 62.17 dm = _____ mm

Change the following units of metric volume:

5. 1.64 mL = _____ dL   6. 0.47 dL = _____ L

7. 10 L = _____ cL   8. 56.9 cL = _____ mL

Change the following units of metric weight:

9. 35.6 mg = _____ g   10. 0.3 g = _____ cg

11. 0.05 g = _____ mg   12. 93 cg = _____ mg

13. 100 mcg = _____ mg   14. 2 mg = _____ mcg

15. 1.0 mcg = _____ mg   16. 7 kg = _____ g

Perform the following miscellaneous conversions:

17. 4 mg = _____ mcg   18. 13 kg = _____ g

19. 2.5 L = _____ mL   20. 0.6 mg = _____ mcg

21. 0.08 g = _____ mg   22. 0.01 mg = _____ mcg

23. 60 mg = _____ g   24. 10.5 mg = _____ mcg

25. 0.5 mL = _____ L   26. 100 mg = _____ dg

27. 3.5 dg = _____ g   28. 3.4 mg = _____ g

29. 30 mg = _____ mcg   30. 13 cg = _____ g

31. 2 kg = _____ g   32. 18 L = _____ mL

33. 450 g = _____ mg   34. 40 mcg = _____ mg

35. 8 L = _____ dL   36. 10 L = _____ cL

37. 46 g = _____ dg   38. 0.5 g = _____ mg

39. 500 mL = _____ L   40. 25 kg = _____ g

*Write the following, using Roman numerals
and symbols:*

41. 3 grains _____   42. 5 drams _____

43. 5 grains _____   44. 10 minims _____

45. 20½ minims _____   46. 5 pints _____

Solve the following:

47. 8 quarts = _____ gallon(s)

48. 4 drams = _____ ounce(s)

49. 2 tablespoons = _____ ounce(s)

50. gr xxx = _____ gram(s)

51. 4 pints = _____ quart(s)

52. 4 ounces = _____ pint(s)

53. 15 grams = _____ dram(s)

54. 12 ounces = _____ teacup(s)

55. 3 glasses = _____ ounces

56. 6 tablespoons = _____ ounce(s)

57. 2 teaspoons = _____ drops

58. 3 tablespoons = _____ teaspoons

59. 2 cups = _____ ounces

60. 8 ounces = _____ pint(s)

thePoint. Additional practice problems to enhance learning and facilitate chapter comprehension can be found at **http://thePoint.lww.com/Boyer8e.**

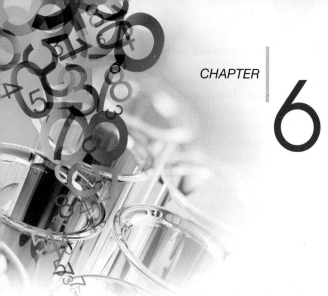

Approximate Equivalents and System Conversions

LEARNING OBJECTIVES

After completing this chapter, you should be able to:

- Identify volume and weight equivalents for the metric and apothecary systems, as well as for household measurements.
- Identify linear equivalents for household measures and the metric system.
- Convert approximate equivalents between the metric, apothecary and household measurement systems.
- Apply three methods of converting between systems: conversion factor, ratio and proportion, and dimensional analysis.

*I*n the preceding chapter, you learned how to change units from one measurement to another *within the same system*. Frequently, you will have to *convert between systems*. When converting, you work with *approximate equivalents* because exact measurements across different systems are not possible. It is essential that you memorize common equivalents and conversions.

A common example of such a discrepancy is between the metric and apothecary systems. For example, a medication label will indicate 5 gr, and its equivalent dosage may be written as 300 mg or 325 mg. Both dosages are correct; the equivalent values are approximate. Remember: Most dosage calculations use 60 mg = 1 gr.

Because you will have to convert between systems, a table of equivalent values is provided. You must memorize the equivalents found in Table 6.1. Remember that when calculating dosages, division is carried out to two decimal places and decimals are rounded off to ensure accuracy (Appendix B).

The metric and English household equivalents for length are rarely used for drug dosage calculations but can be used when applying a paste, cream, or ointment that needs to cover a certain area. However, both are used for linear measurements; for example, to measure wound size, head circumference, abdominal girth, and height.

Dosage Calculations: Converting Between Systems

Whenever the physician orders a drug in a unit that *is in a different system from the drug that is available*,

Table 6.1 **Commonly Used Approximate Equivalents: Metric, Apothecary, and Household Systems of Measure**

Metric	Apothecary	Household
—	1 gtt = 1 m (minim)	1 drop
4 mL	1 dram	—
5 mL	—	1 teaspoon (tsp)
15 mL	4 drams	1 tablespoon (tbsp)
30 mL	8 drams	2 tbsp (1 oz)
180 mL	—	1 teacup (6 oz)
240 mL	—	1 glass/measuring cup (8 oz)
500 mL	1 pt	1 pt (16 oz) = 2 cups
1,000 mL (1 L)	1 qt	1 qt (32 oz) = 4 cups
60–65 mg	1 gr	—
1 g (1,000 mg)	15 gr	—
1 kg (1,000 g)	—	2.2 lb
1 mg = 1,000 mcg	—	—
2.5 cm	—	1 inch

convert to the available system. You want to work in the system of the drug that you have on hand.

RULE

Whenever the desired and available drug doses are in two different systems: Choose the equivalent value and solve for *x*. Always change the desired quantity to the available quantity.

You can use one of three methods to convert between systems: the conversion factor method, ratio and proportion, or dimensional analysis. With each method you must first remember the equivalent value!

The Conversion Factor: Use the equivalent value and either *multiply* (going from a larger to a smaller unit) or *divide* (going from a smaller to a larger unit).

EXAMPLE:

A physician ordered gr $1\frac{1}{2}$ of a medication. You need to give _____ mg.

Equivalent value: 1 gr = 60 mg

Move from a larger unit (grain) to a smaller unit (milligram). Multiply by the conversion factor (60 mg).

$$\text{gr } 1\frac{1}{2} \times 60 = \frac{3}{{}_1 2} \times \frac{\cancel{60}^{\,30}}{1} = 90 \text{ mg}$$

ANSWER: 90 mg

Ratio and Proportion: Select the equivalent value and then set up the proportion using either a colon or fraction format.

EXAMPLE: #1

Give 1.5 ounces of an elixir that is available in mL.

• Change ounces to mL. Choose the equivalent value.

$$30 \text{ mL} = 1 \text{ ounce}$$

• Complete the proportion. Write down what you know. A fraction format is used here.

$$\frac{30 \text{ mL}}{1 \text{ oz}} = \frac{x \text{ mL}}{1.5 \text{ oz}}$$

• Solve for x:

$$x = 30 \times 1.5 = 45 \text{ mL}$$

ANSWER: 45 mL

EXAMPLE: #2   Give gr 1/4 of a drug that is available in mg.

- Select the approximate equivalent value and convert to the system that you have available.

> Change gr 1/4 to mg
> (mg are available).

- Choose the equivalent value.

> 60 mg = 1 gr

- Complete the proportion. Write down *what you know*. A colon format is used here.

> 60 mg : 1 gr :: x mg : gr 1/4
> $x = 60 \times 1/4$

- Solve for x:

$$^{15}\cancel{60} \times \frac{1}{\cancel{4}_1} = 15, \quad x = 15 \text{ mg}$$

ANSWER: 15 mg

Dimensional Analysis: This is presented in detail in Chapter 8.

PRACTICE PROBLEMS

Complete the following. Solve for x or the unknown by using a fraction or colon format.

1. 12 oz = _____ mL

2. 0.3 mL = _____ L

3. 30 mL = _____ tbsp

4. 45 mg = _____ gr

5. 2 tsp = _____ mL

6. 30 kg = _____ lbs

Complete the following. Solve for x or the unknown by using a fraction or colon format.

7. gr 1/200 = _____ mg

8. 3 pt = _____ mL

9. 30 gr = _____ g

10. 300 mcg = _____ mg

11. 30 mL = _____ oz

12. 4 tbsp = _____ mL

13. 6 mg = _____ gr

14. 3 g = _____ gr

15. 1 L = _____ qt

16. 2 qt = _____ L

17. 2.2 lb = _____ kg

18. $\overline{ss}$ oz = _____ mL

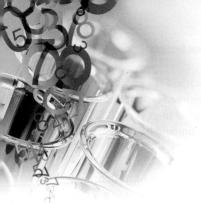

Complete the following. Solve for x by using a fraction or colon format.

1. A child who weighs 55 lb weighs _____ kg.

2. Two (2) grams of Metamucil powder is equivalent to _____ gr.

3. A patient is restricted to four 8-ounce glasses of water per day or _____ mL per day.

4. A patient's abdominal wound measures 10 cm in diameter. The nurse knows that this is equivalent to _____ inch(es).

5. A child was prescribed 10 mL of cough syrup four times a day, as needed. The child's mother administered _____ tsp each time the medication was given.

6. The nurse administered aspirin gr v. She knew this was equivalent to _____ mg.

7. The nurse instilled 3 minims of an eye drop into the patient's right eye, three times per day. The nurse knew that 3 minims were equal to _____ gtt.

8. The physician prescribed 0.4 mg of atropine sulfate to be administered intramuscularly. The medication was labeled in gr per mL. The nurse knew to look for an ampule labeled _____ gr per mL.

9. A patient was to take 2 tbsp of milk of magnesia. Because a medicine cup was available, he poured the milk of magnesia up to the _____-ounce calibration line.

10. A 40-lb child was ordered a drug to be given at 10 mg per kg of body weight. The child weighs _____ kg and should receive _____ mg of the drug.

11. A woman was prescribed 60 mg of a daily vitamin. Her cumulative monthly dose (30 days) would be about _____ g.

12. A patient who takes 1 tbsp of Kayexalate four times per day would be receiving a daily dose equivalent to _____ ounces.

13. A patient takes a 500-mg tablet three to four times per day. He is advised not to exceed a daily dose of 3 g or _____ tablets.

14. A patient is to receive 250 mg of a liquid medication, three times daily. The medicine is available in oral suspension, 250 mg per 5 mL. The nurse should give _____ tsp for each dose.

15. A patient is to receive a 200-mg tablet every 12 hours. The tablet is available in 200-mg quantities. The patient would receive _____ g per day.

16. A child is prescribed a 250-mg tablet every 6 hours. The nurse gives two tablets, four times a day. Each dose would be _____ mg for a daily total dosage of _____ g.

17. A renal patient whose daily fluid intake is restricted to 1,200 mL per day is prescribed eight oral medications, three times daily. The nurse restricts the water needed for swallowing the medications so the patient can have fluids with his meals. The patient is allowed 5 ounces of water, three times a day, with his medications. Therefore, the patient has _____ mL with his drugs.

18. Tylenol liquid is available as 325 mg per 5 mL. A patient who is prescribed 650 mg would be given _____ tsp.

19. A patient is to receive 30 mg of a drug available as 10 mg per teaspoon. The nurse would give _____ tablespoon(s).

20. A physician prescribes 0.3 mg of a drug, twice daily. The medication is available in 0.15-mg tablets. The nurse would give _____ tablets each dose, equivalent to _____ mg daily.

the Point. Additional practice problems to enhance learning and facilitate chapter comprehension can be found at **http://thePoint.lww.com/Boyer8e.**

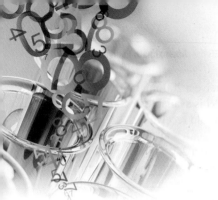

Convert each item to its equivalent value.

1. 0.080 g = _____ mg

2. 3.2 L = _____ mL

3. 1,500 mcg = _____ mg

4. 0.125 mg = _____ mcg

5. 20 kg = _____ g

6. 5 mg = _____ g

7. 155 lb = _____ kg

8. 30 minims = _____ gtt

9. 15 grains = _____ gram(s)

10. 1/2 qt = _____ ounces

11. 3 pt = _____ quart(s)

12. 8 drams = _____ ounce(s)

13. 1 tbsp = _____ tsp

14. 6 tsp = _____ ounce(s)

15. 1 teacup = _____ ounces

16. 2 tbsp = _____ ounce(s)

17. gr $\overline{ss}$ = _____ mg

18. 30 g = _____ ounce(s)

19. 1 oz = _____ mL

20. gr 1 = _____ mg

21. 3 tsp = _____ mL

22. 20 kg = _____ lb

23. gr 1/150 = _____ mg

24. 0.3 mg = _____ gr

25. 1.8 oz = _____ mL

26. 20 mL = _____ tsp

27. 8.5 g = _____ mg

28. 950 mg = _____ g

29. 15 mg = _____ gr

30. 6 mg = _____ mcg

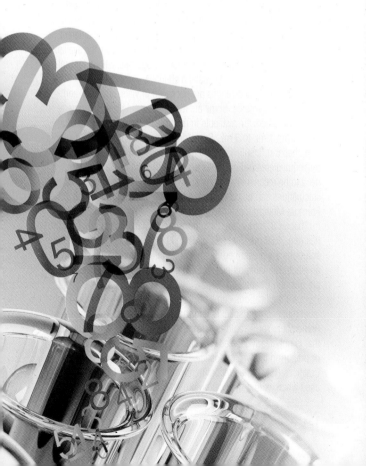

Dosage | 3
Calculations

*A*ccurate dosage calculations are an essential component of the nursing role in the safe administration of medications. Medications are prescribed by their generic (official) name or trade (brand) name and are usually packaged in an average unit dose. Oral medications contain a solid concentration of drug, per quantity of one. Liquid medications contain a specific amount of drug, usually gram weight, dissolved in solution (e.g., mL)—for example, Demerol, 50 mg per mL, or Vistaril, 25 mg per 5 mL. Medication orders refer to drug dosages, so calculations will be necessary if a dosage prescribed is different (with regard to system and/or unit of measurement) from the available dosage. This unit will present common dosage calculations for oral and parenteral routes for adults and children.

Parenteral medications are packaged in vials, ampules, and premeasured syringes. Some are available as single-dose preparations, and others are available in multiple doses. Dosages usually range from 1 mL to 3 mL. Some drugs are measured in units (e.g., heparin, insulin, penicillin), some are found in solutions as milliequivalents (mEq; grams per 1 mL of solution), and others need to be reconstituted from a powder. Oral and parenteral dosage calculations can be completed using ratio and proportion, the Formula Method, or dimensional analysis, which will be introduced in Chapter 8. Intravenous solutions are available in various quantities (e.g., 250 mL, 500 mL, and 1,000 mL). Critical care intravenous solutions are prescribed in smaller quantities and administered via an electronic infusion pump. Examples of these dosage calculations are given in Chapter 11.

All medications come packaged and are clearly labeled. Each label must contain specific information, as outlined in Chapter 7. Remember: You should never prepare or administer any medication that is not clearly labeled. To minimize the possibility or obtaining or preparing the wrong dosage, the Institute for Safe Medication Practices (ISMP) has recommended that the slash line (/) not be used when writing medication orders. Although not universally implemented, some institutions are starting to enforce this recommendation. Therefore, you will notice that the slash is not used in this text or in word problems. However, due to the necessity of brevity for this handbook, the slash line is used within calculations. You can read further about this recommendation at http://www.ismp.org.

Infants and children cannot receive the same dose of medication as adults because a child's physiologic immaturity influences how a drug is absorbed, excreted, distributed, and used. Therefore, pediatric dosages are based on age, body weight, or body surface area. If you are going to give pediatric drugs, you must become familiar with the rules for calculating pediatric dosages, which are given in Chapter 14. Refer to Appendix I for nursing concerns for pediatric drug administration. The older adult also responds differently in the metabolism of medications. See Appendix K for nursing concerns for geriatric drug administration. Appendix J suggests nursing considerations for critical care drug administration.

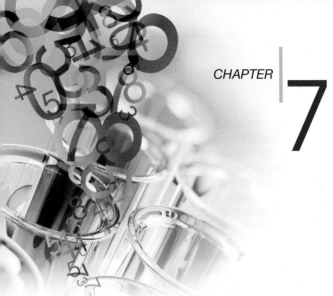

Medication Labels

After completing this chapter, you should be able to:

- Identify a drug's generic and trade name on a medication label.
- Identify drug dosage strength, form, and quantity on a medication label.
- Interpret drug administration requirements and precautions on a medication label.
- Interpret drug manufacturing information on a medication label.
- Interpret drug reconstitution or mixing directions on a medication label.
- Recognize when drug dosage calculations, including equivalent conversions, are necessary—for example, when the prescribed dose is different than the available dose.

*T*o prepare the correct medication that is pre-scribed, you must be able to accurately read a drug label and be familiar with major key points presented in this chapter. Several drug labels will be depicted as examples, and sample drug problems will be presented.

Reading and Interpreting a Drug Label

Some labels are easy to read because they contain a limited amount of information—for example, labels for unit-dose preparation where each tablet or capsule is separately packaged. This is the most common type of label that you will see in a hospital setting. Other labels indicate multiple tablets or capsules, with the dosage of each drug clearly visible. You should be able to recognize the following information on a medication label.

- **Drug name:** Medications are prescribed by their trade or generic name. Drug labels contain *essential and comprehensive* information for the safe administration of medications.
- **Generic or official name:** This is the name given by the company that first manufactures the drug. It appears in smaller letters, sometimes in parentheses, under the brand name. However, because many physicians are now ordering by generic name, labeling is changing to show the generic name in uppercase letters and bolded (e.g., **ATROPINE, MEPERIDINE**).

A drug has only one chemical name, but it may have many different trade names. As a cost-control effort, some insurance companies are now requiring that pharmacists offer a generic brand first, unless contraindicated by the physician.

- **Trade, brand, or proprietary name:** This is the commercial or marketing name that the pharmaceutical company gives a drug. It is printed in bold, large, or capital letters on the label. The ® identifies manufacturer ownership. The drug may be manufactured and marketed by several companies, each using its own trade name.

    If a trade name is followed by ™ it means that the trade name is trademarked and cannot be used by another manufacturer.

- **Drug dosage and strength:** This is the amount of drug available by weight per unit of measure (e.g., Nexium, 40-mg capsules; Demerol, 50 mg per mL). Sometimes the dosage is expressed in two systems (e.g., Nitrostat 0.4 mg [1/150 gr]). Dosage strength is indicated in a solid form (e.g., g, mg, mEq, mcg), in a solid form within a liquid (e.g., mg per mL), in solutions (e.g., 1:1,000), in units (e.g., 1,000 units per mL), or in other preparations such as ointments or patches (e.g., 1% in 0.5 oz).

    Examine the drug label for multiple doses. For example, for Coreg (see Figure 7.1), each of the 100 tablets contains 12.5 mg of the solid drug carvedilol. The usual dose of 12.5 mg per day to 25 mg per day means that a patient may receive 1 to 2 tablets daily.

- **Drug form:** This refers to the form in which the drug is prepared by the manufacturer—for example, tablets, capsules, injectables, oral suspensions,

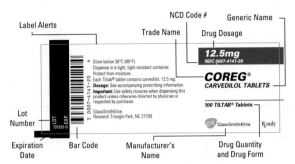

FIGURE 7.1   Coreg. (Courtesy of GlaxoSmithKline, Philadelphia, PA.)

suppositories, ointments, and patches. Some drugs are prepared in several forms. The drug label may also indicate specific characteristics of the drug's form—for example, sustained release (SR), controlled release (CR), long acting (LA), and double strength (DS).

- **Drug quantity:** This is the total amount of the drug in the container (e.g., 100 tablets, 30 capsules, 10 mL) or the total amount of liquid available after reconstitution (e.g., 5 mL, 50 mL). See Figure 7.2, which shows the drug label for Augmentin. When the powder is reconstituted with 47 mL of water, each 5 mL of liquid contains 200 mg of the drug.
- **Drug route of administration:** The route may be indicated on the label, such as oral, sublingual, IM, IV, SC, rectal, topical, otic, and so on. The label will also indicate single- or multiple-use vials, or doses expressed as a ratio or percent (e.g., lidocaine 2%).

Parenteral preparation labels indicate dosages in a variety of ways: percentage and ratio strengths, milliequivalents (number of grams in 1 mL of a solution), 100 units per mL (insulin dosages), and powdered forms that have reconstitution directions. See Figure 7.3, which presents the drug label for Ancef. Each vial contains approximately 330 mg per mL (IM use) after the addition of 2 mL of sterile water.

- **Drug reconstitution or mixing:** As shown in Figures 7.2 and 7.3, the directions for mixing and reconstitution are clear on the drug labels. *Always follow these directions* to ensure the accuracy of drug preparation.
- **Drug manufacturing information:** By federal law, drug labels must contain the following information: **manufacturer name, expiration or volume date, control numbers, a National Drug Code (NDC) number** that is different for every drug, **a bar code** (used for a drug distribution system), and a code identifying one of two official national lists of approved drugs: **USP (United States Pharmacopeia) and NF (National Formulary).** These are identified in Figure 7.1.
- **Drug precautions:** Drug labels also contain precautions about storage and protection from light. For example: Septra tablets (store at 59°F to 77°F in a dry place), heparin (store at controlled room temperature [59°F to 86°F]), promethazine HCl (protect from light and keep covered in the carton until time of use), and Coreg (protect from moisture). Expiration dates indicate the last date that the drug should be used. *Never give a drug beyond its expiration date!*

PRACTICE PROBLEMS

Fill in the blanks for the following questions, referring to the respective medication labels.

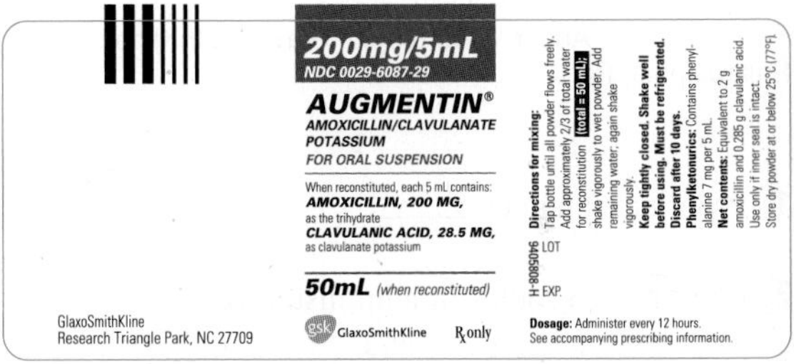

200mg/5mL
NDC 0029-6087-29

AUGMENTIN®
AMOXICILLIN/CLAVULANATE
POTASSIUM
FOR ORAL SUSPENSION

When reconstituted, each 5 mL contains:
AMOXICILLIN, 200 MG,
as the trihydrate
CLAVULANIC ACID, 28.5 MG,
as clavulanate potassium

50mL *(when reconstituted)*

GlaxoSmithKline
Research Triangle Park, NC 27709

GlaxoSmithKline   ℞ only

Directions for mixing: Tap bottle until all powder flows freely. Add approximately 2/3 of total water for reconstitution (total = 90 mL); shake vigorously to wet powder. Add remaining water; again shake vigorously.
Keep tightly closed. Shake well before using. Must be refrigerated. Discard after 10 days.
Net contents: Equivalent to 2 g amoxicillin and 0.285 g clavulanic acid.
Phenylketonurics: Contains phenylalanine 7 mg per 5 mL.
Use only if inner seal is intact.
Store dry powder at or below 25°C (77°F).

H-9095096 LOT
H- EXP.

Dosage: Administer every 12 hours.
See accompanying prescribing information.

FIGURE 7.2 Augmentin. (Courtesy of GlaxoSmithKline, Philadelphia, PA.)

1. Generic name: _____

2. Dosage strength: _____

3. Precautions: _____

4. Reconstitute: _____ reconstitution

5. Reconstituted dosage: _____

6. Drug volume after reconstitution: _____

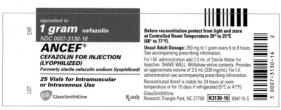

FIGURE 7.3   Ancef. (Courtesy of GlaxoSmithKline, Philadelphia, PA.)

1. Proprietary name: _____

2. Identify two routes of administration:
   _____ and _____

3. Reconstitute: _____

4. Approximate dose per mL after reconstituting:
   _____

5. Usual adult dose: _____

6. Precautions: _____

FIGURE 7.4 Requip. (Courtesy of GlaxoSmithKline, Philadelphia, PA.)

1. Generic name: _____

2. NDC number: _____

3. Dosage strength: _____

4. Drug quantity: _____

5. Drug form: _____

6. Precautions: _____

7. Trade name: _____

8. Manufacturer: _____

Answer each question by referring to the specific drug labels presented in the accompanying figures.

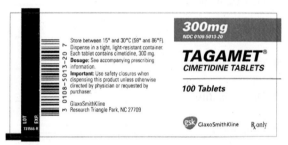

300mg
NDC 0108-5013-20

TAGAMET®
CIMETIDINE TABLETS

100 Tablets

Store between 15° and 30°C (59° and 86°F).
Dispense in a tight, light-resistant container.
Each tablet contains cimetidine, 300 mg.
Dosage: See accompanying prescribing information.
Important: Use safety closures when dispensing this product unless otherwise directed by physician or requested by purchaser.

GlaxoSmithKline
Research Triangle Park, NC 27709

gsk GlaxoSmithKline   R only

LOT
EXP.
731566-R

FIGURE 7.5   Tagamet. (Courtesy of GlaxoSmithKline, Philadelphia, PA.)

1. A physician prescribed 600 mg of Tagamet, twice daily. The nurse would administer _____ tablet(s) for each dose. The patient would receive _____ mg of Tagamet in 24 hr.

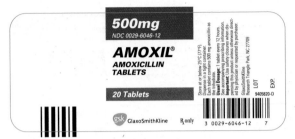

FIGURE 7.6   Amoxil. (Courtesy of GlaxoSmithKline, Philadelphia, PA.)

2. A patient is to receive 2 g of amoxicillin (Amoxil) every 24 hr for 10 days. The medication is given every 6 hr. The patient would receive _____ mg or _____ tablet(s) for each dose.

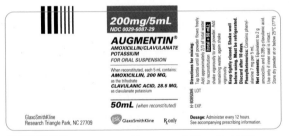

FIGURE 7.7   Augmentin. (Courtesy of GlaxoSmithKline, Philadelphia, PA.)

3. A physician prescribed 100 mg of Augmentin every 8 hr for a 3-year-old. The nurse would administer _____ mL for each dose. The child would receive _____ mg and _____ mL in 24 hr.

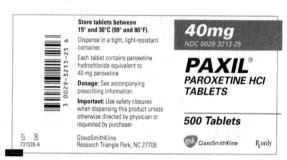

FIGURE 7.8　Paxil. (Courtesy of GlaxoSmithKline, Philadelphia, PA.)

4. A physician prescribed 40 mg of Paxil twice a day. The patient would receive _____ tablet(s) per dose and _____ mg per day.

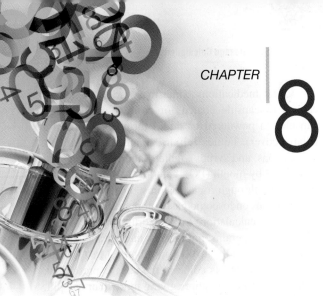

Oral Dosage Calculations

LEARNING OBJECTIVES

After completing this chapter, you should be able to:

- Describe the various types of oral medications.
- Apply *ratio and proportion* to solve oral drug dosage problems.
- Apply the *Formula Method* to solve oral drug dosage problems.
- Apply *dimensional analysis* to solve oral drug dosage problems.
- Solve dosage calculation problems for medications in similar and different measurement systems (use equivalent values when necessary).
- Understand the rationales for critical thinking checks.

Oral medications come in a variety of forms: caplets (a capsule coated for ease of swallowing), capsules (a powdered or liquid form of a drug in a gelatin cover), liquids (elixirs, emulsions, solutions, suspensions, and syrups), tablets, and pills. Drugs are prescribed by mouth (PO), enterally, via a nasogastric (NG) tube, through a gastrostomy tube, or through a percutaneous endoscopic gastrostomy tube (PEG).

Dosage calculations for solid drugs usually involve tablets (grains, grams, milligrams, micrograms); liquid calculations usually involve milliliters. Most tablets, capsules, and caplets come in the dosage prescribed, or the prescription requires giving more than one pill, breaking a scored tablet in half, or crushing and/or mixing a dose when swallowing is difficult. Enteric-coated tablets (a coating that promotes intestinal rather than gastric absorption) and sustained-release (SR), controlled-release (CR), or extended release (XL) tablets should be taken whole. Sublingual tablets are placed under the tongue and absorbed through the circulation.

When the dosage prescribed by the health care provider (physician, nurse practitioner) differs from the available quantity, dosage calculation is required. This chapter will present three methods to solve dosage calculation problems: proportions (using either two ratios [colon format] or two fractions [fraction format]), the Formula Method, and dimensional analysis. Each method requires understanding measurement systems and system equivalencies. Each method of problem solving will be demonstrated, using sample problems. Each section is followed by practice problems. An end-of-chapter review is provided to

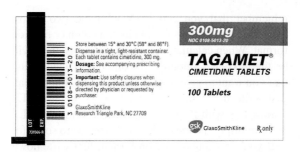

FIGURE 8.1 Tagamet. (Courtesy of GlaxoSmithKline, Philadelphia, PA.)

reinforce the steps of calculation. See Figure 8.1 for an example of an oral drug medication label.

Calculating Oral Dosages

When medications are prescribed and available in the same system (e.g., metric) and the same unit of size (e.g., grains, mcg, mg), dosage calculations are easy. When the prescribed or desired dosage is different from what is available or what "you have" (different systems or different units) you must convert to the same system (usually metric) and the same units (the smaller the better) before calculating dosages. To do this you need to use an equivalent value. When calculating oral dosages, you can use ratio and proportion, the Formula Method, or dimensional analysis.

Ratio and Proportion

Ratio and proportion is explained in detail in Chapter 4. For a quick review here, you need to remember that you can work with the two ratios, expressed as a proportion, in either a colon or fraction format. When calculating dosage problems, the x will be the unknown amount—the amount of medication that you want to give. If you are using a colon format, first write down the known ratio (25 mg : 1 mL). Follow this with the unknown ratio (10 mg : x mL). Then multiply the means by the extremes to solve for x. If you are using a fraction format, first write down the known fraction $\left(\frac{25 \text{ mg}}{1 \text{ mL}}\right)$, followed by the unknown fraction $\left(\frac{10 \text{ mg}}{x \text{ mL}}\right)$. Cross-multiply and then divide both sides of the equation by the number in front of x.

The Formula Method

The Formula Method is a quick way to solve dosage calculations. Always use critical thinking checks to make sure that your answer is logical. Sometimes it will be necessary to convert between systems (use equivalents) before calculating the dosage. Two examples will be provided after the Rule. *The symbol* R_x *is used throughout this book to indicate "desired amount."*

RULE

To apply the Formula Method: the *prescribed* amount of drug becomes the *desired* (D) amount and the numerator of the fraction; the drug that is *available*—the amount that *you have* (H)—becomes the denominator of the fraction; and the drug form (tablet, mL) is the *quantity* (Q) that is multiplied by the terms in the fraction labeled (D/H). The unknown (x) is what you need to calculate to give the medication.

The Formula Method: The Basic Equation:

$$\frac{D \text{ (desired amount)}}{H \text{ (have on hand)}} \times Q \text{ (quantity)}$$

$$= x \text{ (amount to give)}$$

$$\left\{ \frac{D}{H} \times Q = x \right\}$$

D = **desired (prescribed) amount in the given units of measurement**

H = **what you have (available); the dosage strength**

Q = **quantity; drug form (tablet, mL)**

x = **amount to give; the unknown dosage**

EXAMPLE: #1   The physician prescribed 100 mg of a medication that is available as 50-mg tablets.

$$\frac{D \text{ (desired)}}{H \text{ (have)}} \times Q = x \text{ tablets}$$

$$\frac{100 \text{ mg}}{50 \text{ mg}} \times 1 = x$$

$$\frac{\overset{2}{\cancel{100}}}{\underset{1}{\cancel{50}}} \times 1 = x \text{ (use cancellation, then multiplication)}$$

$$x = 2 \times 1 = 2$$

ANSWER: 2 tablets

EXAMPLE: #2   The physician prescribed gr 1/2 of a medication that is available as 15 mg per tablet. Note: Because you have two systems, you need to first convert to the same

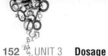
system. Always convert to the system *that is available*! Therefore, for this problem, convert grain to mg. Use the equivalent 60 mg = 1 gr.

60 mg : 1 gr = x mg : gr 1/2

$x = 60 \times 1/2$

$x = 30$ mg

$$\frac{D \text{ (desired)}}{H \text{ (have)}} \times Q = x \text{ tablets}$$

$$\frac{30 \text{ mg}}{15 \text{ mg}} \times 1 = x$$

$$\frac{\overset{2}{\cancel{30}}}{\underset{1}{\cancel{15}}} \times 1 = x \text{ (use cancellation, then mul-}$$
tiplication), $x = 2 \times 1 = 2$

ANSWER: 2 tablets

Dimensional Analysis

Dimensional analysis (DA) is a problem-solving method also known as the unit-factor method or the factor-label method. Dimensional analysis is used frequently in the sciences to solve chemistry equations. Its popularity in nursing is increasing.

Dimensional analysis uses one equation (fraction method), thus minimizing errors and eliminating the need to memorize a formula. *The unit in the denominator of the second fraction must be the same as the unit in the numerator of the first fraction.* Frequently, *conversion factors* (*equivalents*) will be needed if the units are not in the same system. Placement of the units of the fractions is important for multiplication and cancellations to be accurate.

The Basic Terms for Dimensional Analysis:

- **Desired dose:** the dose to be given, *what you desire.* Also known as the given quantity.
- **Wanted quantity:** the answer (x); that is, mL, oz, mg.
- **Available dose:** the available amount of the drug, *what you have.*
- **Units:** the measure of the drug form (tablet, mL).
- **Unit placement or path and cancellation:** placement of the units of the fractions in the numerator and the denominator positions so cancellation can occur.
- **Factors:** dosages in fraction format.
- **Conversion factors:** the *equivalents* used to convert between systems.
- **Computation:** *the calculation process.* Cancel first, multiply the numerators, multiply the denominators, and then divide the product of the numerators by the product of the denominators.

There is more than one way to set up a dimensional analysis equation. You can begin with the *given quantity* (desired dose) or the *wanted quantity* (x). There are four ways to set up the equation. No matter which fraction placement you use, the equation is designed for multiplication and cancellation. Three of the following examples start with the given quantity, and one starts with the wanted quantity. One problem will be used to demonstrate each of the four approaches.

EXAMPLE: Give 120 mg of a drug that is available as gr i per tablet. Use a conversion factor.

Start with the Given Quantity: Use a Vertical Line to Separate the Fractions

$$\frac{120 \text{ mg}}{} \left| \frac{1 \text{ tablet}}{\text{gr i}} \right| \frac{\text{gr i}}{60 \text{ mg}}$$

$$\frac{120 \text{ \cancel{mg}}}{} \left| \frac{1 \text{ tablet}}{\text{\cancel{gr} i}} \right| \frac{\text{\cancel{gr} i}}{60 \text{ \cancel{mg}}}$$

$$= \frac{120 \times 1 \text{ (tablet)} \times 1}{60} = \frac{\cancel{120}^{2}}{\cancel{60}_{1}} = \frac{2}{1} = 2 \text{ tablets}$$

Start with the Given Quantity: Use an x to Separate the Fractions

$$\frac{120 \text{ mg}}{} \times \frac{1 \text{ tablet}}{\text{gr i}} \times \frac{\text{gr i}}{60 \text{ mg}}$$

$$\frac{120 \text{ \cancel{mg}}}{} \times \frac{1 \text{ tablet}}{\text{\cancel{gr} i}} \times \frac{\text{\cancel{gr} i}}{60 \text{ \cancel{mg}}}$$

$$= \frac{120 \times 1 \text{ (tablet)} \times 1}{60}$$

$$= \frac{\cancel{120}^{2}}{\cancel{60}_{1}} = \frac{2}{1} = 2 \text{ tablets}$$

Start with the Given Quantity: Use an = Sign to Separate the Fractions

$$\frac{120 \text{ mg}}{} = \frac{1 \text{ tablet}}{\text{gr i}} = \frac{\text{gr i}}{60 \text{ mg}}$$

$$\frac{120 \text{ \cancel{mg}}}{} = \frac{1 \text{ tablet}}{\text{\cancel{gr} i}} = \frac{\text{\cancel{gr} i}}{60 \text{ \cancel{mg}}}$$

$$= \frac{120 \times 1 \text{ (tablet)} \times 1}{60} = \frac{\cancel{120}^{2}}{\cancel{60}_{1}}$$

$$= \frac{2}{1} = 2 \text{ tablets}$$

Start with the Wanted Quantity: Use an = Sign After the x

$$x \text{ tablets(s)} = \frac{1 \text{ tablet}}{\cancel{\text{gr}} \text{ i}} \times \frac{120 \cancel{\text{ mg}}}{60 \cancel{\text{ mg}}} \times \cancel{\text{gr}} \text{ i}$$

$$= \frac{120 \times 1 \text{ (tablet)} \times 1}{60} = \frac{\cancel{120}^{2}}{\cancel{60}_{1}} = \frac{2}{1}$$

$$= 2 \text{ tablets}$$

Note: For this book, dimensional analysis equations will *begin with the given quantity*. Use an x to separate the fractions.

RULE

To apply the dimensional analysis formula: Follow the steps in the following example.

EXAMPLE: Give 250 mg of a drug. The drug is available as 500 mg per tablet.

- Write down *what you desire* (250 mg). This given quantity will be the numerator of the first fraction.

    250 mg

- Write down *what you have available* (500 mg per tablet) as the second fraction. Placement of the units must be set up to allow for cancellation. The denominator of the second fraction must be in the same units as the numerator of the first fraction.

$$\frac{250 \text{ mg}}{} \times \frac{1 \text{ tablet}}{500 \text{ mg}} =$$

- Cancel the opposite and matching units of measure in the denominators and numerators. The remaining measure (tablet) is what is desired. Complete the mathematical calculations.

$$\frac{250 \text{ mg}}{} \times \frac{1 \text{ tablet}}{500 \text{ mg}} = x$$

$$\frac{250 \cancel{\text{ mg}}}{} = \frac{1 \text{ tablet}}{500 \cancel{\text{ mg}}} = \frac{250 \times 1 \text{ (tablet)}}{500}$$

$$= \frac{\cancel{250}^{1}}{\cancel{500}_{2}} = \frac{1}{2} = \frac{1}{2} \text{ tablet}$$

ANSWER: $\frac{1}{2}$ tablet

R U L E

To apply the dimensional analysis formula using a conversion factor (equivalent): Follow the steps in the following example.

EXAMPLE: Give 0.5 g of a drug. The medication is available as 250 mg per tablet.

- Write down *what you desire* (0.5 g). This given quantity will be the numerator of the first fraction.

    0.5 g

- Write down *what you have available* (250 mg per tablet) as the second fraction.

    $$0.5 \text{ g} \times \frac{1 \text{ tablet}}{250 \text{ mg}}$$

- A conversion factor is needed because the units are not the same. The equivalent value is 1 g = 1,000 mg. Cancel the opposite and matching units of measure in the denominators and numerators. The remaining measure (tablet) is what is desired. Complete the mathematical calculations.

$$\frac{0.5 \text{ g}}{250 \text{ mg}} \times \frac{1 \text{ tablet}}{} = \frac{1{,}000 \text{ mg}}{1 \text{ g}}$$

$$= \frac{0.5 \times 1 \text{ (tablet)} \times 1{,}000}{250} = \frac{\overset{2}{\cancel{500}}}{\underset{1}{\cancel{250}}}$$

$$= \frac{2}{1} = 2 \text{ tablets}$$

ANSWER: 2 tablets

Dosage Calculations for Medications in the Same System and the Same Unit of Measurement

RULE

When the desired and available drug doses are different but in the same system and same unit of measurement: Use one of the following three methods to calculate dosages.

For this chapter, the _colon format will be used when working with ratio and proportion._ You can also use the fraction format if you wish.

EXAMPLE #1:　R_x: 0.250 mg
Have: 0.125-mg tablet
Give: _____ tablet(s)
This sample problem will be solved using all three methods.

Ratio and Proportion

0.125 mg : 1 tablet = 0.250 mg : x
$0.125x = 0.250$

$$x = \frac{\cancel{0.250}^{2}}{\cancel{0.125}_{1}} = \frac{2}{1} = 2 \text{ tablets}$$

ANSWER: 2 tablets

The Formula Method

$$\frac{D}{H} \times Q = x$$

$$\frac{0.250}{0.125} \times x = \frac{\cancel{0.250}^{2}}{\cancel{0.125}_{1}} = \frac{2}{1} = 2 \text{ tablets}$$

ANSWER: 2 tablets

Dimensional Analysis

$$\frac{0.250 \text{ mg}}{} \times \frac{1 \text{ tablet}}{0.125 \text{ mg}}$$

$$= \frac{0.250 \cancel{\text{ mg}}}{} \times \frac{1 \text{ tablet}}{0.125 \cancel{\text{ mg}}}$$

$$= \frac{0.250 \times 1 \text{ (tablet)}}{0.125}$$

$$= \frac{\cancel{250}^{2}}{\cancel{125}_{1}} = \frac{2}{1} = 2 \text{ tablets}$$

ANSWER: 2 tablets

EXAMPLE #2:   R$_X$: gr 1/2 p.r.n.

Have: gr 1/4 per tablet

Give: _____ tablet(s)

Ratio and Proportion

gr 1/4 : 1 tablet = gr 1/2 : x tablets

$1/4x = 1/2$

$$x = \frac{\frac{1}{2}}{\frac{1}{4}} = \frac{1}{\cancel{2}_1} \times \frac{\cancel{4}^2}{1} = 2 \text{ tablets}$$

Answer: 2 tablets

The Formula Method

$$\frac{D}{H} \times Q = x$$

$$\frac{\text{gr } \frac{1}{2}}{\text{gr } \frac{1}{4}} = \frac{1}{\cancel{2}_1} \times \frac{\cancel{4}^2}{1} = \frac{2}{1} = 2 \text{ tablets}$$

Answer: 2 tablets

Dimensional Analysis

$$\frac{\text{gr } \frac{1}{2}}{\text{gr } \frac{1}{4}} \times 1 \text{ tablet}$$

$$= \frac{\cancel{\text{gr}} \frac{1}{2}}{\cancel{\text{gr}} \frac{1}{4}} \times \frac{1 \text{ tablet}}{1} = \frac{\frac{1}{2} \times 1 \text{ (tablet)}}{\frac{1}{4}}$$

$$= \frac{\frac{1}{2}}{\frac{1}{4}} = \frac{1}{\cancel{2}_1} \times \frac{\cancel{4}^2}{1} = \frac{2}{1} = 2 \text{ tablets}$$

Answer: 2 tablets

EXAMPLE #3: R_x: 100 mg
Have: 20 mg per 5 mL
Give: _____ mL

Ratio and Proportion

20 mg : 5 mL = 100 mg: x
$20x = 500$

$$x = \frac{500}{20} = \frac{\cancel{50}^{25}}{\cancel{2}_1} = 25 \text{ mL}$$

ANSWER: 25 mL

The Formula Method

$$\frac{D}{H} \times Q = x$$

$$\frac{100 \text{ mg}}{20 \text{ mg}} \times 5 = \frac{500}{20} = \frac{\cancel{50}^{25}}{\cancel{2}_1} = 25 \text{ mL}$$

ANSWER: 25 mL

Dimensional Analysis

$$\frac{100 \text{ mg}}{} \times \frac{5 \text{ mL}}{20 \text{ mg}}$$

$$= \frac{100 \ \cancel{\text{mg}}}{} \times \frac{5 \text{ mL}}{20 \ \cancel{\text{mg}}} = \frac{100 \times 5 \ (\text{mL})}{20}$$

$$= \frac{\cancel{500}^{50}}{\cancel{20}_2} = \frac{\cancel{50}^{25}}{\cancel{2}_1} = 25 \text{ mL}$$

ANSWER: 25 mL

Dosage Calculations for Medications in the Same System but with Different Units of Measurement

RULE

When the desired and available drug doses are in the same system but different units of measurement: Convert to like units, change to the smaller unit, and use one of the three methods to calculate dosages.

EXAMPLE #1: Rx: 4 g daily
Have: 500 mg per tablet
Give: _____ tablet(s)

CONVERT TO LIKE UNITS:
To convert 4 g to mg, move the decimal point (4.0 g) three places to the right: 4,000.
Then 4 g = 4,000 mg

Ratio and Proportion

500 mg : 1 tablet = 4,000 mg : x
$500x = 4,000$

$$x = \frac{4,000}{500} = \frac{\cancel{40}^{\,8}}{\cancel{5}_{1}} = 8 \text{ tablets}$$

ANSWER: 8 tablets

The Formula Method

$$\frac{D}{H} \times Q = x$$

$$\frac{4,000 \text{ mg}}{500 \text{ mg}} \times 1 = x$$

$$\frac{4,000}{500} = \frac{\cancel{40}^{8}}{\cancel{5}_{1}} = 8 \text{ tablets}$$

ANSWER: 8 tablets

Dimensional Analysis

$$\frac{4 \text{ g}}{500 \text{ mg}} \times \frac{1 \text{ tablet}}{} = \frac{1,000 \text{ mg}}{1 \text{ g}}$$

$$= \frac{4 \cancel{\text{ g}}}{500 \cancel{\text{ mg}}} \times \frac{1 \text{ (tablet)}}{} = \frac{1,000 \cancel{\text{ mg}}}{1 \cancel{\text{ g}}}$$

$$= \frac{4 \times 1 \text{ (tablet)} \times 1,000}{500 \times 1} = \frac{\overset{40}{\cancel{4,000}}}{\cancel{500}_{5}} = \frac{40}{5} = 8 \text{ tablets}$$

ANSWER: 8 tablets

EXAMPLE #2: R: 1.2 g in two equally divided doses
Have: 600 mg per tablet
Give: _____ tablet(s)

CONVERT TO
LIKE UNITS: To convert 1.2 g to mg, move the decimal point (1.2 g) three places to the right: 1,200.
Then 1.2 g = 1,200 mg

Ratio and Proportion

600 mg : 1 tablet = 1,200 mg : x
$600x = 1,200$

$$x = \frac{\cancel{1,200}^{2}}{_{1}\cancel{600}} = 2 \text{ tablets}$$

> **ANSWER:** 2 tablets in 2 divided doses
> or 1 tablet each dose

The Formula Method

$$\frac{D}{H} \times Q = x$$

$$\frac{1,200 \text{ mg}}{600 \text{ mg}} \times 1 = x$$

$$\frac{\cancel{1,200}^{2} \cancel{\text{mg}}}{_{1}\cancel{600} \cancel{\text{mg}}} = \frac{2}{1} = 2 \text{ tablets}$$

> **ANSWER:** 2 tablets in two divided doses
> or 1 tablet each dose

Dimensional Analysis

$$\frac{1.2 \text{ g}}{} \times \frac{1 \text{ tablet}}{600 \text{ mg}} = \frac{1,000 \text{ mg}}{1 \text{ g}}$$

$$= \frac{1.2 \cancel{\text{ g}}}{} \times \frac{1 \text{ (tablet)}}{600 \cancel{\text{ mg}}} = \frac{1,000 \cancel{\text{ mg}}}{1 \cancel{\text{ g}}}$$

$$= \frac{1.2 \times 1 \text{ (tablet)} \times 1,000}{600 \times 1} = \frac{\cancel{1,200}^{2}}{_{1}\cancel{600}}$$

$$= \frac{2}{1} = 2 \text{ tablets}$$

> **ANSWER:** 2 tablets in divided doses
> or 1 tablet each dose

Dosage Calculations for Medications in Different Systems

_R U L E_

When the desired and available drug doses are in different systems: Convert to the available system, select the equivalent value, write down what you know in a fraction or colon format, and use ratio and proportion or the Formula Method to calculate dosages. Use a conversion factor for dimensional analysis.

EXAMPLE:	R_x: morphine sulfate gr 1/4 Have: morphine sulfate 10-mg tablets Give: _____ tablet(s) To use ratio and proportion, use the equivalent and convert to the available system.
CONVERT TO SAME SYSTEM:	Milligrams are *available*. Change gr 1/4 to mg. *Equivalent*: 1 gr = 60 mg
COMPLETE THE PROPORTION:	1 gr : 60 mg = 1/4 gr : x mg $x = 1/4 \times 60$
SOLVE FOR X:	$\dfrac{1}{4} \times 60 = 15$ $x = 15$ mg

Ratio and Proportion

10 mg : 1 tablet = 15 mg : x
10x = 15

$$x = \frac{\cancel{15}^{3}}{\cancel{10}_{2}} = \frac{3}{2} = 1\frac{1}{2} \text{ tablets}$$

ANSWER: 1½ tablets

The Formula Method

$$\frac{D}{H} \times Q = x$$

$$\frac{15 \text{ mg}}{10 \text{ mg}} \times 1 = x$$

$$x = \frac{\overset{3}{\cancel{15}} \text{ mg}}{\underset{1}{\cancel{10}} \text{ mg}} = \frac{3}{2} = 1\frac{1}{2} \text{ tablets}$$

ANSWER: 1½ tablets

Dimensional Analysis

$$\frac{\text{gr } \frac{1}{4} \times \frac{1 \text{ tablet}}{10 \text{ mg}}}{} = \frac{60 \text{ mg}}{\text{gr } 1}$$

$$= \frac{\cancel{\text{gr}} \frac{1}{4} \times \frac{1 \text{ tablet}}{10 \cancel{\text{mg}}}}{} = \frac{60 \cancel{\text{mg}}}{\cancel{\text{gr}} 1}$$

$$= \frac{\frac{1}{4} \times 1 \, (\text{tablet}) \times 60}{10 \times 1} = \frac{\overset{3}{\cancel{15}}}{\underset{2}{\cancel{10}}}$$

$$= \frac{3}{2} = 1\frac{1}{2} \text{ tablets}$$

ANSWER: 1½ tablets

PRACTICE PROBLEMS

1. R$_X$:   160 mg daily
   Have: 40-mg tablets
   Give _____ tablet(s).

2. R$_X$:   1,500 mg
   Have: 500 mg per 5 mL
   Give _____ mL.

3. R$_X$:   150 mg
   Have: 300-mg tablets
   Give _____ tablet(s).

4. R$_X$:   20 mg
   Have: 10 mg per 5 mL
   Give _____ mL.

5. R$_X$:   7.5 mg t.i.d.
   Have: 2.5-mg tablets
   Give _____ tablet(s), t.i.d.

6. R$_X$:   100 mg every 4 to 6 hr, as needed
   Have: 50-mg tablets
   Give _____ tablet(s) for each dose.

7. R$_X$:   75 mg
   Have: 15 mg per mL
   Give _____ mL.

8. R$_X$:   25 mg
   Have: 50-mg tablets
   Give _____ tablet(s).

9. R$_x$:   4 g to be taken in four equally divided
             doses
    Have: 500-mg tablets
    Give _____ tablet(s) each dose.

Critical Thinking Check

Refer to question 9. If 5 g were ordered in five
divided doses, does it seem logical that one
500-mg tablet would be given? _____ **Yes or
No?**

---

10. R$_x$:   0.5 g every 8 hr
    Have: 250 mg per teaspoon
    Give _____ mL.

Critical Thinking Check

Refer to question 10. Since the suspension was
ordered every 8 hr, does it seem logical that the
patient should be awakened during the night for
his medication? _____ **Yes or No?**

---

11. A medication is on hand in a syrup (2 mg per mL).
    The prescribed dose is 3 teaspoons. Give _____
    mL, which would be equal to _____ mg.

12. A drug is on hand in a liquid as 250 mg per 5 mL.
    The initial dose of 125 mg for 3 days requires
    giving _____ teaspoon(s) each day for a total
    of _____ mL over 3 days.

13. A medication is on hand in a transdermal patch containing 0.0015 g. The system delivers 0.5 mg over 72 hr. After 72 hr, _____ mg remain.

14. A physician prescribed 20 mg of syrup to be administered every 4 hr for pain. The drug was available as 50 mg per 5 mL. The nurse should give _____ mL q4h.

15. A physician prescribed 0.8 g of a liquid medication. The drug was available in a strength of 200 mg per mL. The nurse should give _____ mL.

16. A physician prescribed 60 mg of a diuretic. The mediation was available as 15 mg per tablet. The nurse should give _____ tablets.

17. A physician prescribed 0.4 mg of a medication for nutritional deficiency. The medication was available as 0.6 mg per mL. The nurse should administer _____ mL.

18. A physician prescribed 200 mcg of a medication for vertigo. The drug was available as 0.6 mg per mL. The nurse should give _____ mL.

19. The physician prescribed 7.5 mg of a drug, once daily. The medication was available as 2.5-mg tablets. The nurse should give _____ tablets.

20. The physician prescribed 100 mg of a drug that was available in 40-mg tablets. The nurse should give _____ tablets.

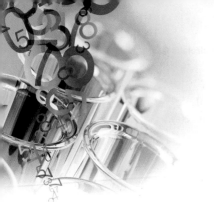

End of Chapter Review

Solve the following problems:

1. R$_x$:   30 mg daily
   Have: 10-mg tablets
   Give _____ tablet(s).

2. R$_x$:   300 mg
   Have: 100-mg tablets
   Give _____ tablet(s).

3. R$_x$:   1.5 g daily
   Have: 250 mg per 5 mL
   Give _____ mL.

4. R$_x$:   0.2 g
   Have: 50-mg tablets
   Give _____ tablet(s).

5. R$_x$:   gr 1/200
   Have: 0.3-mg tablets
   Give _____ tablet(s).

6. R$_x$:   gr 1/2
   Have: 15-mg tablets
   Give _____ tablet(s).

7. R_x: 20 g
   Have: 30 g in 45 mL
   Give _____ ounce(s).

8. R_x: gr 1/150
   Have: 0.4-mg tablets
   Give _____ tablet(s).

9. R_x: gr 1/4
   Have: 10 mg per 5 mL
   Give _____ mL.

10. R_x: 0.1 g
    Have: 100-mg tablets
    Give _____ tablet(s).

11. R_x: gr 1/4 four times a day
    Have: 15-mg tablets
    Give _____ tablet(s) per dose for a total
    of _____ tablet(s) daily.

12. R_x: 5 mg
    Have: 1.25-mg tablets
    Give _____ tablet(s).

13. R_x: 100 mg q.i.d.
    Have: 10 mg per mL
    Give _____ teaspoon(s) for each dose.

14. R_x: 1.5 g daily in three equal doses, 500 mg
    per tablet. The tablet is available as
    500 mg. The nurse would give _____
    mg, three times a day.

15. R$_x$:   2.4 g daily for rheumatoid arthritis
Have: 600-mg tablets
Give _____ tablet(s) a day.

16. R$_x$:   10 mg daily, every 6 hr, for 2 weeks
Have: 2.5-mg tablets
Give _____ tablets daily, equally divided
over 6 hr.

Critical Thinking Check

Refer to question 16. If the drug was ordered
q.i.d. rather than every 6 hr, would you expect
the patient to receive the same number of pills in
24 hr? _____ **Yes or No?**

---

17. R$_x$:   500 mg
Have: 0.25 g per 5 mL
Give _____ mL or _____ teaspoon(s).

Critical Thinking Check

Refer to question 17. Does it seem logical that
1 g of the drug could also be prescribed based
on the available dosage? _____ **Yes or No?**

---

thePoint. Additional practice problems to enhance
learning and facilitate chapter comprehension can be
found on **http://thePoint.lww.com/Boyer8e.**

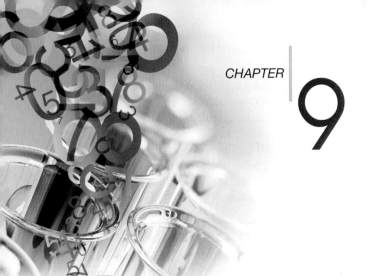

Parenteral Dosage Calculations

LEARNING OBJECTIVES

After completing this chapter, you should be able to:

- Define the term *parenteral* as it refers to medication administration.
- Distinguish among three types of parenteral injection: intradermal, subcutaneous, and intramuscular.
- Identify the parts of a syringe.
- Distinguish among the different types of syringes: hypodermic, tuberculin, U-100, and U-50 insulin.
- Describe the differences in needles (length, gauge, and use).
- Explain how parenteral medications are supplied (ampules, vials, and prefilled cartridges and syringes).
- Interpret a parenteral drug label.
- Calculate parenteral medication dosages using ratio and proportion, the Formula Method, and dimensional analysis.

*T*he term *parenteral* refers to any route of drug delivery other than gastrointestinal. It is used when the oral route would be ineffective (delayed absorption time, drug interactions, or patient's inability to swallow) or the drug needs to be quickly absorbed. Medications can be administered intramuscularly (IM), subcutaneously (SQ), intradermally (ID), and intravenously (IV). Remember: Needle *precautions must always be followed* when administering parenteral medications.

Insulin is covered in Chapter 12 and heparin in Chapter 13. Intravenous therapies, including IV piggyback (IVPB) and IV push, are covered in Chapters 10, 11, and 14. Pediatric calculations are covered in Chapter 14. Reconstitution of powders for injections is presented in Chapter 15.

Packaging, Syringes, and Needles

Packaging. Parenteral medications are commonly supplied in liquid or solution form and packaged in ampules (small, glass, sealed containers that hold a single dose), vials (small, glass or plastic bottles with a rubber tip and cover), or in prefilled cartridges and syringes that contain a single drug dose. Preparations that come in a powder form must be reconstituted according to the manufacturer's directions.

Syringes. There are three kinds of syringes: hypodermic, tuberculin, and insulin (U-100 and U-50, low dose). Syringes have three parts: a barrel with milliliter (mL) calibrations, a plunger, and a tip. Luer-Lok syringes have a tip that syringe-specific needles twist into; non–Luer-Lok syringes have a tip that needles

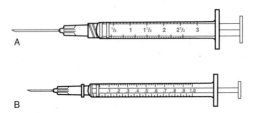

FIGURE 9.1 A. Standard 3-mL Luer-Lok syringe.
B. Tuberculin syringe.

slip into. Some syringes have a safety glide (which covers the needle after use), whereas others are needleless (IV use). See Figure 9.1 for an example of a standard, 3-mL, Luer-Lok hypodermic syringe and a 1-mL tuberculin syringe; a picture of a needless port is given in Appendix L.

Hypodermic and Tuberculin Syringes. The standard, 3-mL syringe is marked on one side in 0.1-mL increments, with longer lines indicating 0.5 mL and 1.0 mL. Smaller syringes still indicate minims but are not used frequently, to avoid errors. Most injectable medications are given in a 3-mL syringe unless the dosage can easily be measured in a 1-mL syringe. Markings on the 1-mL narrow tuberculin syringe (commonly used for solutions less than 1 mL) can be found in tenths (0.1 mL) and hundredths (0.01 mL). It is essential that you read these calibrations accurately so that you give the correct amount of medication. When checking the liquid medication in the syringe, always remember to (a) hold the syringe *at eye level*, (b) draw the medication into the barrel, and (c) use the *top of the black ring* to measure the correct amount. See Figures 9.2 and 9.3 for examples of labels for two different parenteral drug preparations.

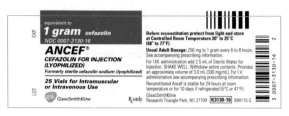

FIGURE 9.2 Ancef. (Courtesy of GlaxoSmithKline, Philadelphia, PA.)

Insulin syringes. Insulin syringes are only used for insulin! Insulin, supplied in quantities of 100 units per mL, is administered using a U-100 syringe (up to 1-mL volume, marked every 2 units) or a U-50, low-dose syringe (up to 0.5-mL volume, marked every 1 unit), which is no longer used very often in the hospital. It is used in home care. A U-30 syringe is being phased out but may be used in the home. Two insulin syringes are shown in Figure 12.3

Needles. Needles are distinguished by their length (inches) and their gauge (width or diameter) and have different uses. The lower the gauge number, the larger is the diameter. For example, a 14-gauge IV needle has a larger diameter than a 27-gauge needle

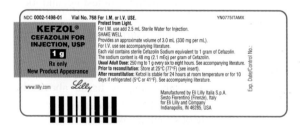

FIGURE 9.3 Kefzol. (Courtesy of Eli Lilly Company, Indianapolis, IN.)

Table 9.1 **Needle Gauge and Length for Different Types of Injection**

Type of Injection	Needle Gauge	Needle Length (inches)
Intradermal	25	3/8 to 5/8
Intramuscular	18 to 23	1 to 3
Intravenous	14 to 25	1 to 3
Subcutaneous	23 to 28	5/8 to 7/8

used for intradermal injections. See Table 9.1 for an example.

Types of Injections

- **Intradermal Injections:** into the dermis (under the outer layer of skin or epidermis). Refer to the picture Administering an Intradermal Injection, in Appendix D.

  The intradermal route is used for:
  1. Small amounts of drugs (0.1 mL to 0.5 mL). The average dose is 0.1 mL.
  2. Solutions that are nonirritating and slowly absorbed.
  3. Allergy testing, tuberculin skin testing, and local anesthesia.
  4. Common sites: inner surface of forearm and upper back below the scapula.

- **Subcutaneous Injections:** under the skin or dermis into the fibrous, subcutaneous tissue above the muscle. Refer to Appendix E.

  The subcutaneous route is used for:
  1. Small amounts of drugs (0.5 mL to 1 mL).
  2. Insulin

3. Heparin
4. Tetanus toxoid

• **Intramuscular Injections:** into the body of a striated muscle. Refer to the picture Administering an Intramuscular Injection, in Appendix F.

   The intramuscular route is used for:

1. Drugs that require a rapid rate of absorption.
2. Drugs that would be ineffectively absorbed in the gastrointestinal tract.
3. Drugs that are given in large volume.

Dosage Calculations for Medications in the Same System and the Same Unit of Measurement

To calculate parenteral dosage problems, follow the same rules that you used for oral dosage calculations, using one of the three calculation methods. Ratio and proportion, the Formula Method, or dimensional analysis can be used. Remember to follow any guidelines regarding patient age, weight, or special considerations before administering parenteral medications.

_R U L E_

Whenever the prescribed or desired and available drug dosages are different but in the same system and the same unit of measurement: Use one of three methods to calculate dosages. Refer to Chapter 8 for a quick review of these three methods.

EXAMPLE #1: R_x: 1 mg
Have: 5 mg per mL
Give: _____ mL

Ratio and Proportion

5 mg : 1 mL = 1 mg : x mL
$5x = 1$

$$x = \frac{1}{5} \times 1 \text{ mL} = 0.2 \text{ mL}$$

ANSWER: 0.2 mL

The Formula Method

$$\frac{D}{H} \times Q = x$$

$$\frac{1 \text{ mg}}{5 \text{ mg}} \times 1 = x$$

$$\frac{1}{5} \times 1 \text{ mL} = 0.2 \text{ mL}$$

ANSWER: 0.2 mL

Dimensional Analysis

$$1 \text{ mg} \times \frac{1 \text{ mL}}{5 \text{ mg}}$$

$$\frac{1 \; \cancel{\text{mg}}}{} \times \frac{1 \text{ mL}}{5 \; \cancel{\text{mg}}} = \frac{1 \times 1 \text{ (mL)}}{5}$$

$$= \frac{1}{5} = 0.2 \text{ mL}$$

ANSWER: 0.2 mL

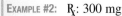

EXAMPLE #2: R$_x$: 300 mg
Have: 150 mg per mL
Give: _____ mL

Ratio and Proportion

150 mg : 1 mL = 300 mg : x mL
150x = 300

$$x = \frac{\cancel{300}^{\,2}}{\cancel{150}_{\,1}} = \frac{2}{1} = 2 \text{ mL}$$

ANSWER: 2 mL

The Formula Method

$$\frac{D}{H} \times Q = x$$

$$\frac{300}{150} \times 1 = x$$

$$\frac{\cancel{300}^{\,2}}{\cancel{150}_{\,1}} = \frac{2}{1} \times 1 \text{ mL} = 2 \text{ mL}$$

ANSWER: 2 mL

Dimensional Analysis

$$\frac{300 \text{ mg}}{} \times \frac{1 \text{ mL}}{150 \text{ mg}}$$

$$= \frac{300 \ \cancel{\text{mg}}}{} \times \frac{1 \text{ mL}}{150 \ \cancel{\text{mg}}} = \frac{300 \times 1 \ (\text{mL})}{150}$$

$$= \frac{\cancel{300}^{\,2}}{\cancel{150}_{\,1}} = \frac{2}{1} = 2$$

ANSWER: 2 mL

EXAMPLE #3:   R$_x$: 35 mg
                     Have: 50 mg per mL
                     Give: _____ mL

Ratio and Proportion

50 mg : 1 mL = 35 mg : x
$50x = 35$

$$x = \frac{\overset{7}{\cancel{35}}}{\underset{10}{\cancel{50}}} = \frac{7}{10} = 0.7 \text{ mL}$$

ANSWER: 0.7 mL

Formula Method

$$\frac{D}{H} \times Q = x$$

$$\frac{35}{50} \times 1 = x$$

$$\frac{\overset{7}{\cancel{35}}}{\underset{10}{\cancel{50}}} = \frac{7}{10} \times 1 \text{ mL} = 0.7 \text{ mL}$$

ANSWER: 0.7 mL

Dimensional Analysis

$$\frac{35 \text{ mg}}{} \times \frac{1 \text{ mL}}{50 \text{ mg}}$$

$$= \frac{35 \cancel{\text{ mg}}}{} \times \frac{1 \text{ mL}}{50 \cancel{\text{ mg}}} = \frac{35 \times 1 \text{ (mL)}}{50}$$

$$= \frac{\overset{7}{\cancel{35}}}{\underset{10}{\cancel{50}}} = \frac{7}{10} = 0.7$$

ANSWER: 0.7 mL

Dosage Calculations for Medications in the Same System but Having Different Units of Measurement

RULE

Whenever the prescribed or desired and available drug dosages are in the same system but in different units of measurement: Convert to like units, change to the smaller unit, and use one of three methods to calculate dosages. Remember to use a conversion factor if you use dimensional analysis.

| EXAMPLE: | R̥: 0.25 mg
Have: 500 mcg per 2 mL
Give: _____ mL |

| CONVERT TO LIKE UNITS: | To convert 0.25 mg to mcg, move the decimal point (0.25 mg) three places to the right. Then 0.25 mg = 250 mcg. |

Ratio and Proportion

500 mcg : 2 mL = 250 mcg : x mL
$500x = 500(250 \times 2)$

$$x = \frac{\cancel{500}^{1}}{\cancel{500}^{1}} = 1 \text{ mL}$$

ANSWER: 1 mL

The Formula Method

$$\frac{D}{H} \times Q = x$$

$$\frac{250}{500} \times 2 = x$$

$$\frac{\cancel{250}^{1} \text{ mcg}}{\cancel{500}^{2} \text{ mcg}} = \frac{1}{2} \times 2 \text{ mL} = 1 \text{ mL}$$

ANSWER: 1 mL

Dimensional Analysis

$$\frac{0.25 \text{ mg}}{} \times \frac{2 \text{ mL}}{500 \text{ mcg}}$$

$$= \frac{0.25 \cancel{\text{mg}}}{} \times \frac{2 \text{ mL}}{500 \cancel{\text{mcg}}} = \frac{1,000 \cancel{\text{mcg}}}{1 \cancel{\text{mg}}}$$

$$= \frac{0.25 \times 2 \, (\text{mL}) \times 1,000}{500 \times 1} = \frac{\cancel{500}^{1}}{\cancel{500}_{1}} = 1 \text{ mL}$$

ANSWER: 1 mL

Dosage Calculations for Medications in Different Systems

RULE

Whenever the prescribed or desired and available drug dosages are in different systems: Convert to the same system (use available system), select the equivalent value, write down what you know in a fraction or ratio format, and use ratio and proportion to solve for *x*. Use one of three methods to calculate dosages. Use a conversion factor if you are using dimensional analysis.

EXAMPLE: R_x: gr 1½ IM, b.i.d.
Have: 60 mg per mL
Give: _____ mL, b.i.d.

EQUIVALENT: gr 1 = 60 mg

COMPLETE THE PROPORTION: $gr\ 1 : 60\ mg = gr\ 1\frac{1}{2} : x\ mg$

SOLVE FOR x: $1x = 1\frac{1}{2} \times 60$

$$x = \frac{3}{2_1} \times \cancel{60}^{\,30} = 90\ mg$$

Ratio and Proportion

60 mg : 1 mL = 90 mg : x mL
$60x = 90$

$$x = \frac{\cancel{90}^{\,3}}{\cancel{60}_2} = \frac{3}{2} = 1.5\ mL$$

ANSWER: 1.5 mL

The Formula Method

$$\frac{D}{H} \times Q = x$$

$$\frac{90}{60} \times 1 = x$$

$$\frac{\cancel{90}^{\,3}}{\cancel{60}_2} = \frac{3}{2} = 1.5\ mL$$

ANSWER: 1.5 mL

Dimensional Analysis

$$\frac{gr\ 1.5}{} \times \frac{1\ mL}{60\ mg}$$

$$= \frac{\cancel{gr}\ 1.5}{} \times \frac{1\ mL}{60\ \cancel{mg}} = \frac{60\ \cancel{mg}}{\cancel{gr}\ 1}$$

$$= \frac{1.5 \times 1\ (mL) \times 60}{60 \times 1}$$

$$= \frac{\cancel{90}^{\ 3}}{\cancel{60}_{\ 2}} = 1.5\ mL$$

ANSWER: 1.5 mL

Penicillin

Penicillin is one of a limited number of medications that is available in units per mL as well as mg per mL. Insulin (covered in Chapter 12) and heparin (covered in Chapter 13) are two other common medications that you will need to become familiar with. When calculating dosages for penicillin, you can use ratio and proportion, the Formula Method, or dimensional analysis.

RULE

To prepare penicillin for injection: Check the prescribed or desired units to be given, and use one of three methods to calculate dosages.

EXAMPLE: A patient is prescribed 300,000 units of penicillin G procaine to be administered every 12 hr (q12h). Penicillin G procaine is available as 600,000 units per 1.2 mL.

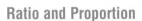

Ratio and Proportion

600,000 units : 1.2 mL = 300,000 : x mL
600,000x = 300,000 × 1.2
600,000x = 360,000

$$x = \frac{\cancel{360,000}^{36}}{\cancel{600,000}_{60}} = \frac{\cancel{36}^{6}}{\cancel{60}_{10}} = \frac{6}{10} = 0.6 \text{ mL}$$

ANSWER: 0.6 mL

The Formula Method

$$\frac{D}{H} \times Q = x$$

$$\frac{\cancel{300,000}^{3}}{\cancel{600,000}_{6}} = \frac{\cancel{3}^{1}}{\cancel{6}_{2}} = \frac{1}{2}$$

$$\frac{1}{2} \times 1.2 \text{ mL} = 0.6 \text{ mL}$$

ANSWER: 0.6 mL

Dimensional Analysis

$$\frac{300,000 \text{ units}}{} = \frac{1.2 \text{ mL}}{600,000 \text{ units}}$$

$$\frac{300,000 \ \cancel{\text{units}}}{} = \frac{1.2 \ (\text{mL})}{600,000 \ \cancel{\text{units}}}$$

$$= \frac{300,000 \times 1.2}{600,000} = \frac{\cancel{360,000}^{36}}{\cancel{600,000}_{60}}$$

$$= \frac{\cancel{36}^{6}}{\cancel{60}_{10}} = \frac{6}{10} = 0.6 \text{ mL}$$

ANSWER: 0.6 mL

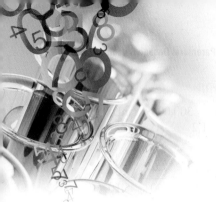

Complete the following problems:

1. Give 0.002 g of a drug, IM, per day, for 5 days, for severe intestinal malabsorption. The injection is on hand as 1.0 mg per mL. The nurse should give _____ mL a day for 5 days.

2. Give 60 mg of a diuretic IM in three equally divided doses every 8 hr for 2 days. The drug is available for injection as 10 mg per mL. The nurse should give _____ mL every 8 hr.

3. Give 0.3 g of a drug that is available as 100 mg per mL for injection. The nurse should give _____ mL.

4. Give 10 mg of a drug that is available as 5 mg per mL. The nurse should draw up _____ mL.

5. Give 4 mg of a drug that is available as 5 mg per mL. The nurse should give _____ mL.

6. Give 2 mg of a drug, p.r.n., every 4 to 6 hr. The medication is available as 5 mg per mL. The nurse should give _____ mL every 4 to 6 hours as needed.

7. The physician requested that a patient receive 1.5 mg of a drug, IM, every 3 to 4 hr as needed for pain. The medication is available for injection as 2.0 mg per mL. The nurse should give _____ mL every 3 to 4 hr, p.r.n.

8. Give 35 mg, IM, of a drug that is available for injection as 50 mg per mL. The nurse should give _____ mL.

9. Give 6 mg of a drug, weekly. The medication is available as 2 mg per mL. The nurse should give _____ mL every week.

10. Give 3 mg, IM, of a drug preoperatively to induce drowsiness. The drug is available as 5 mg per mL. The nurse should give _____ mL.

11. Give 1 mg of a drug every 4 to 6 hr for analgesia. The drug is available as 4 mg per mL. The nurse should give _____ mL every 4 to 6 hr.

12. Give 30 mg of a diuretic. The drug is available as 40 mg per mL. The nurse should give _____ mL.

13. Give 0.5 mg of a medication that is available in a vial as gr 1/150 per 1.0 mL. The nurse should give _____ mL.

14. Give 50 mg of a medication that is available in vials containing gr i per mL. The nurse should give _____ mL.

15 Give gr 1/5, IM, every 4 to 6 hr for severe pain.
The medication is available as 15 mg per mL.
The nurse should give _____ mL, every 4 to 6 hr,
as needed.

Critical Thinking Check

Because the available medication strength
(15 mg per mL) is a stronger drug concentration
than the prescribed medication (gr 1/5), does it
seem logical that greater than 1 mL would be
given? _____ **Yes or No?**

---

16 Give 6 mg of a drug. The medication is available
as 10 mg per mL for injection. The nurse should
give _____ mL.

17. Give 0.15 mg IM of a drug that is available as
0.2 mg per mL. The nurse should give _____ mL.

18. Give 25 mg, IM, of a drug preoperatively. The
drug is available as 100 mg per 2 mL. The nurse
should give _____ mL.

19. Give 50 mg, q6h, of a drug that is available as
25 mg per mL. The nurse should give _____ mL.

20. Give 0.1 mg of a drug, IM, prior to an operative
procedure. The drug is available as 50 mcg per
mL. The nurse should give _____ mL.

21. Give 500 mcg, IM, of a drug that is available as
1 mg per mL. The nurse should give _____ mL.

22. Give 30 mg, of a drug that is available as 20 mg per mL. The nurse should give _____ mL.

23. Give 0.25 mg of a drug that is available as 250 mcg per mL. The nurse should give _____ mL.

24. Give 4 mg, IM, of a drug that is available as 2 mg per mL. The nurse should give _____ mL.

25. Give gr 1/4, q6h, of a drug that is available as 30 mg per mL. The nurse should give _____ mL.

26. Give 90 mg of a drug, IV, q6h, that is available as 120 mg per 2 mL. Give _____ mL.

27. Give 0.05 mg of a drug that is available as 100 mcg per 5 mL. Give _____ mL.

28. Give 0.4 g of a drug that is available as 500 mg per 5 mL. Give _____ mL.

29. Give 250 mg of a drug that is available as 0.75 grams per 3 mL. Give _____ mL.

30. The physician prescribed Crysticillin 600,000 units, IM, as a single dose. Crysticillin is available in a 12-mL vial labeled 500,000 units per mL. The nurse should give _____ mL.

31. The physician prescribed 300,000 units of Bicillin, IM, q12h for 5 days. Bicillin is packaged as 600,000 units per mL. The nurse should give _____ mL per dose.

32. The physician prescribed penicillin G potassium 125,000 units, IM, q12h. The medication is available in solution as 250,000 units per mL. The nurse should give _____ mL every 12 hr.

33. Penicillin G benzathine 1.2 million units was prescribed, IM, as a single injection. The drug is available as 300,000 Units per mL. The nurse should give _____ mL.

Critical Thinking Check

Would it seem logical to give a dosage of 1.2 M units as a single injection? _____ **Yes or No?**

---

thePoint Additional practice problems to enhance learning and facilitate chapter comprehension can be found on **http://thePoint.lww.com/Boyer8e.**

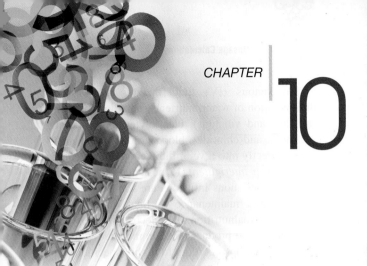

Intravenous Therapy

LEARNING OBJECTIVES

After completing this chapter, you should be able to:

- Explain the purpose of intravenous therapy (fluids and medicine).
- Identify various infusion sets and tubing.
- Distinguish among infusion pumps, syringe pumps, and a patient-controlled analgesia (PCA) pump.
- Calculate infusion time in hours and minutes.
- Calculate flow rate in milliliters per hour (mL per hr) for gravity and pump infusion.
- Calculate rate of infusion of an intravenous (IV) push.
- Calculate flow in mL per hr for manual and electronic regulation when the infusion is *less than 1 hr.*
- Calculate flow rate in drops per minute (gtt per min) using the Standard Formula and dimensional analysis.
- Calculate flow rate using the Quick Formula with a constant factor.
- Describe intermittent intravenous fluid therapy (IV piggyback [IVPB] and IV push).

*I*ntravenous (IV) fluid therapy involves the administration of water, nutrients (e.g., dextrose, protein, fats, and vitamins), electrolytes (e.g., sodium, potassium, and chloride), blood products, and medications directly into a vein. Intravenous fluids can be *continuous or intermittent* (IV push and IV piggyback [IVPB]). Continuous infusions are for fluid replacement or fluid maintenance to treat disorders like dehydration, malnutrition, and electrolyte imbalance. Blood and blood products are administered with special Y-type tubing according to highly specific protocols and institutional requirements.

Parenteral nutrition is nutritional supplementation given IV when the oral or enteral route cannot be used. Parenteral nutrition is given through a central venous access device (TPN) or a peripheral line (PPN). The same principles guiding IV therapy are used for parenteral therapy. Enteral tube feeding via a pump is covered in Chapter 15.

This chapter will discuss the basic information about types of equipment, fluids, and infusion calculations (drop factors, drip rates, flow rates, and infusion time). Special IV calculations used in critical care situations are treated in Chapter 11.

Key Terms

- **Drip rate:** the number of drops entering the drip chamber based on the size of the IV tubing (gtt per min).
- **Drop factor:** the size of the drop entering the drip chamber based on the size of the IV tubing.

Drop factors range from 10 gtt per mL to 60 gtt per mL.
- **Flow rate:** the rate in mL per hr given over time.
- **Infusion time:** the time in hours and minutes that it takes for an IV to completely infuse.
- **Titration:** adjustment of the IV medication dosage within prescribed parameters to achieve a desired effect.

Intravenous Fluids

A physician's order for intravenous fluid therapy *must include* the name and amount of the IV solution, any medication that should be added, and the time period for infusion (e.g., q8h, at 50 mL per hr, or in terms of mcg/kg/min, mcg/kg/hr, or mg per min) for critical care. The physician's order is usually written as mL per hr to be infused (flow rate). The flow rate is regulated manually by straight gravity, by volume control, or via an electronic infusion device.

Intravenous fluids are prepared in sterile, plastic bags (most common) or glass bottles, and the quantity of solution ranges from 50 mL to 1,000 mL. Solutions are clearly labeled.

Standard abbreviations are used for the type and concentration of IV solutions: D (dextrose), NS (normal saline), RL (Ringer's lactate), S (saline), and W (water). Numbers refer to the percentage of the solution strength. For example, D5W refers to 5% dextrose (solute) dissolved in a water solution (usually 500 mL to 1,000 mL). Normal saline is a 0.9% sodium chloride solution (900 mg per 100 mL). Percentages less than 0.9% are equivalent to 1/3 (0.33%) or 1/2

(0.45%). Ringer's lactate is an isotonic solution that replenishes fluids and electrolytes.

Review the types of IV fluids and abbreviations in Table 10.1 and interpret the following sample physician orders:

- Administer 1,000 mL of D5W at 125 mL per hr.
- Administer 1,000 mL of 0.9% NS every 12 hr for 2 days.

Table 10.1 **Commonly Prescribed Intravenous Fluids**

Fluid	Abbreviation
0.9% Sodium chloride solution	NS
0.45% Sodium chloride solution	1/2 NS
0.25% Sodium chloride solution	1/4 NS
5% Dextrose in water	5% D/W
	D5W
10% Dextrose in water	10% D/W
	D10W
5% Dextrose in 0.45% sodium chloride solution	D5 1/2NS
Dextrose with Ringer's lactate solution	D/RL
Lactated Ringer's solution	RL
Plasma volume expanders	
Dextran	
Albumin	
Hyperalimentation	
Total parenteral nutrition	TPN
Partial parenteral nutrition	PPN
Fat emulsions	
Intralipid	

- Administer 500 mL of D10W at 83 mL per hr.
- Administer 100 mL of RL over 4 hr at 25 mL per hr.

Intravenous Infusion Sets and Lines

Intravenous fluids are administered via an IV infusion set. The set consists of IV fluids in a sterile, plastic bag or glass bottle connected by IV tubing. An IV set includes a drip chamber with spike, one or more injection ports (access for IVPB and IVP drugs), a filter, and a slide or roller clamp used to regulate the drops per minute. The *primary* IV line is either a *peripheral* line, usually inserted into the arm or hand, or a *central* line, inserted into a large vein in the chest (subclavian) or neck (jugular). *Secondary* IV lines, also known as IV piggyback (IVPB), are used for intermittent, smaller-quantity infusions (e.g., a medication in 50 mL to 100 mL of fluid) and are attached to the primary line through an injection port. A *peripherally inserted central catheter* (PICC line) is threaded into the superior vena cava through a vein in the arm.

Infusion Devices

IV fluids can be regulated by several different electronic infusion devices: pumps, syringe pumps, patient-controlled analgesia (PCA) pumps, and a balloon device used in home care. Infusion pumps are used when small amounts of fluids/medications must be given over a strictly regulated period of time. The *infusion pump* consistently exerts pressure against the resistance of the tubing or the fluid at a prese-lected rate. Pumps are not gravity dependent! A pump delivers a set quantity (mL per hr); however, pumps can be dangerous because they continue to infuse even in the presence of infiltration or phlebi-tis. Infusion pumps can also regulate IVPB infusions by overriding the primary IV line. There are standard pumps and more complex ones that are used for spe-cialty units.

A *syringe pump* (a syringe filled with medication and attached to a pump) regulates medications that must be given at a very low rate over 5 min to 20 min. A *PCA pump,* used by patients for pain management (the patient pushes a control button to self-administer the medication), delivers a set amount of a narcotic in a prefilled syringe over a specified time period. As a safety measure, there is a time interval when no medication can be delivered even if the patient pushes the button. The RN is responsible for the PCA load-ing dose, the narcotic injector vial, and the pump setting.

To set an electronic infusion pump, you must enter the quantity of fluid to be given (mL) and the milliliters per hour (mL per hr). To set a pump used in critical care units, you also enter information such as medication name, dosage concentration, fluid quan-tity, and the patent's weight. The medication may also be titrated to the patient's blood pressure.

Infusion pumps are used whenever possible. However, when IVs are administered by gravity flow, you need to know the drop factor (drops per milliliter) in order to calculate the drip rate (gtt per min). See Figure 10.1.

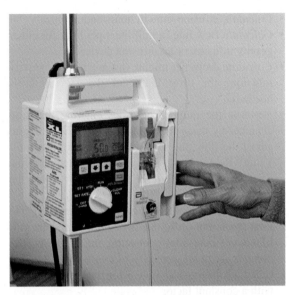

FIGURE 10.1 Electronic infusion pump. (From Taylor, C., Lillis, C., LeMone, P., and Lynn, P. [2008]. *Fundamentals of nursing. The art and science of nursing care* [6th ed.]. Philadelphia: Lippincott Williams & Wilkins.)

Calculate Intravenous Fluid Administration

The physician's IV order *always includes* the quantity of solution (mL) to be given and the time period, either in hours (e.g., q8h, q12h) or in terms of amount (e.g., 100 mL per hr). The nurse is responsible for regulating the infusion either by gravity or programming the milliliters per hour on the pump. The remainder of this chapter will cover what you need to know to:

- *Calculate* infusion time in hours and minutes.
- *Calculate* flow rate in milliliters per hour for either gravity infusion or an infusion device.
- *Calculate* drops per minute (gtt per min) for gravity infusion (the drop factor of the IV tubing is needed).
- *Regulate* the number of drops entering the drop chamber by using the roller clamp on the tubing to adjust the flow rate (count the number of drops for 1 min). Remember to always hold a watch up to the drip chamber at *eye level* to accurately count the drops!
- *Set* the electronic infusion pump by entering the total amount of milliliters to be infused and the milliliters per hour after connecting the IV fluids. *The pump is set in mL per hr.*
- Calculate drops per minute using the Quick Formula with a constant factor.
- Calculate drops per minute for intermittent intravenous infusion.
- Calculate infusion time for an IV push medication.

Calculate Infusion Time in Hours and Minutes

A simple one-step ratio (division) is all that is needed when total volume is known and milliliters per hour have been ordered. *Always round off to the nearest tenth!* Use this formula:

$$\frac{\text{Total volume (mL ordered)}}{\text{Milliliters per hour (mL/hr)}}$$

$$= \text{Number of hours to run}$$

Note: When the number of hours includes additional minutes, you need to round to the nearest tenth. Then multiply the part of an hour by 60 min to get the exact number of minutes.

EXAMPLE #1:   The patient is to receive 1,000 mL of D5W solution at 125 mL per hr.

$$\frac{\text{Total volume}}{\text{mL/hr}} = \text{Number of hours,}$$

$$\frac{1,000 \text{ mL}}{125 \text{ mL/hr}} = \frac{8 \text{ hr}}{1} = 8 \text{ hr}$$

ANSWER: 8 hr

EXAMPLE #2:   The patient is to receive 1,000 mL of NS at 80 mL per hr.

$$\frac{\text{Total volume}}{\text{mL/hr}} = \text{Number of hours,}$$

$$\frac{1,000 \text{ mL}}{80 \text{ mL/hr}} = \frac{12.5 \text{ hr}}{1} = 12.5 \text{ hr}$$

ANSWER: 12½ hr, or 12 hr and 30 min
(½ × 60 min = 30 min)

Calculate Flow Rate in Milliliters per Hour for Gravity or Pump Infusions

To calculate milliliters per hour, all you need to know is the total volume to be infused over time. When a pump is used, simply set the infusion rate at milliliters per hour after connecting the IV fluids, and start the infusion.

RULE

To calculate milliliters per hour: Use one of three methods to calculate dosages: ratio and proportion, dimensional analysis, or the Standard Formula (total volume divided by total time in hours), which is basically simple division.
Note: *When the infusion time is less than 1 hr, you need to use total time in minutes. For dimensional analysis, include the conversion factor (60 min) in the calculation.*

EXAMPLE #1: A patient is to receive 1,000 mL of lactated Ringer's solution over a 6-hr period. The patient should receive _____ mL per hr.

Ratio and Proportion

1,000 mL : 6 hr $= x$ mL : 1 hr
$6x = 1,000$

$$x = \frac{1,000}{6}$$

$x = 166.6$ mL per hr

ANSWER: 167 mL per hr

The Standard Formula

$$\frac{\text{Total volume (mL)}}{\text{Total time (hr)}} = \text{mL/hr}$$

$$\frac{1,000}{6} \text{mL} = 166.6 \text{ mL/hr}$$

ANSWER: 167 mL per hr

Dimensional Analysis

Because two factors are already given, all that is necessary is simple division.

The given quantity is 1,000 mL and the wanted quantity (x) is mL per hr.

$$\frac{1,000 \text{ (mL)}}{6 \text{ (hr)}} = \frac{1,000}{6} = 166.6$$

$$\text{or } \frac{167 \text{ mL}}{\text{hr}}$$

ANSWER: 167 mL per hr

EXAMPLE #2:   A patient is to receive 1 g of an antibiotic in 50 mL of NS over 30 min.

Ratio and Proportion

50 mL : 30 min = x mL : 60 min (1 hr)
$30x = 3,000$

$$x = \frac{\cancel{3,000}^{100}}{\cancel{30}_1} = 100 \text{ mL/hr}$$

ANSWER: 100 mL per hr

The Standard Formula

$$\frac{\text{Total volume (mL)}}{\text{Total time (min)}} = \frac{x \text{ (mL/hr)}}{60 \text{ min}}$$

$$\frac{50 \text{ mL}}{30 \text{ min}} = \frac{x \text{ (mL)}}{60 \text{ min}}$$

$$30x = 3,000 \ (50 \times 60)$$

$$x = \frac{\overset{100}{\cancel{3000}}}{\cancel{30}_1} = 100 \text{ mL/hr}$$

ANSWER: 100 mL per hr

Dimensional Analysis

Two factors are already given. You need to include the conversion factor: 60 min = 1 hr.

$$\frac{50 \text{ mL}}{30 \text{ min}} \times \frac{60 \text{ min}}{1 \text{ hr}}$$

$$\frac{50 \text{ (mL)}}{30} \times \frac{60}{1 \text{ (hr)}} = \frac{50 \text{ (mL)} \times 60}{30 \times 1 \text{ (hr)}}$$

$$= \frac{\overset{100}{\cancel{3,000}}}{\cancel{30}_1} = \frac{100}{1} = 100 \text{ mL/hr}$$

ANSWER: 100 mL per hr

Calculate Drip Rate or Drops per Minute

To calculate drops per minute (gtt per min), you need three pieces of information:

- The *total volume* to be infused in milliliters

- The *drop factor* of the tubing you will use

- The *total time* for the infusion *in minutes or hours*

The flow rate of the IV solution as it passes through the drip chamber is determined by the drop

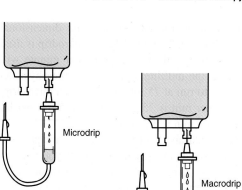

FIGURE 10.2 Left: A drip chamber of an IV tubing for a microdrip (60 gtt/mL). Right: A drip chamber of an IV tubing for a macrodrip (gtt/mL varies).

factor (drops per milliliter) of the tubing set. The drop factor is printed on the IV tubing package. It is either a *macrodrip* (10, 15, or 20 drops per min) or a *microdrip* (60 drops per min). The microdrip contains a needle in the chamber to make the drops smaller. See Figure 10.2 and Table 10.2.

Several formulas and dimensional analysis can be used to calculate flow rate in drops per minute. The

Table 10.2   **Common Drop Factors for IV Tubing Sets**

Macrodrop	10 gtt per mL
	15 gtt per mL
	20 gtt per mL
Microdrop	60 gtt per mL

Standard Formula for gtt per min and dimensional analysis will be used. Note: When a microdrip is used with a drop factor of 60, the drops per minute will always equal the milliliters per hour. If the physician orders an IV to run at 75 mL per hr with a microdrip, then the gtt per min is 75; if it runs at 35 mL per hr, then the gtt per min is 35.

Note: When an IV order includes a medication, usually the drug is already premixed. If you need to add the drug, simply prepare the medication as directed and then calculate the flow rate using one of the following formulas.

The Standard Formula

$$x = \frac{\text{Total volume} \times \text{Drop factor}}{\text{Total time (min)}}$$
$$= \text{Drops per minute (gtt/min)}$$

EXAMPLE #1: Administer 1,000 mL of D5W every 8 hr. The drop factor is 15 gtt per mL.

The Standard Formula

$$\frac{\text{Total volume} \times \text{Drop factor}}{\text{Total time (min)}}$$
$$= \text{Drops per minute}$$

$$\frac{1,000 \text{ mL} \times 15}{480 \text{ min } (60 \times 8)} = \frac{15,000}{480}$$
$$= 31.25 \text{ gtt/min}$$

ANSWER: 31 gtt per min

Dimensional Analysis

$$\frac{\text{Total volume}}{\text{hr}} \times \frac{\text{Drop factor}}{\text{mL}} \times \frac{1 \text{ hr}}{60 \text{ min}}$$

$$\frac{1,000 \text{ mL}}{8 \text{ hr}} \times \frac{15 \text{ gtt}}{1 \text{ mL}} \times \frac{1 \text{ hr}}{60 \text{ min}}$$

$$\frac{1,000 \times 15 \text{ (gtt)} \times 1}{8 \times 1 \times 60 \text{ (min)}}$$

$$= \frac{15,000}{480} = 31.25 \text{ gtt/min}$$

ANSWER: 31 gtt per min

EXAMPLE #2:   Administer 500 mL of 0.9% NS over 6 hr. The drop factor is 20 gtt per mL.

The Standard Formula

$$\frac{\text{Total volume} \times \text{Drop factor}}{\text{Total time (min)}} = \text{gtt/min}$$

$$\frac{500 \text{ mL} \times 20}{360 \text{ min}} = \frac{10,000}{360} = 27.7 \text{ gtt/min}$$

ANSWER: 28 gtt per min

Dimensional Analysis

$$\frac{\text{Total volume}}{\text{hr}} = \frac{\text{Drop factor}}{\text{mL}} = \frac{1 \text{ hr}}{60 \text{ min}}$$

$$\frac{500 \text{ mL}}{6 \text{ hr}} \times \frac{20 \text{ gtt}}{1 \text{ mL}} \times \frac{1 \text{ hr}}{60 \text{ min}}$$

$$\frac{500 \times 20 \text{ (gtt)} \times 1}{6 \times 1 \times 60 \text{ (min)}} = \frac{10,000}{360}$$

$$= 27.7 \text{ gtt/min}$$

ANSWER: 28 gtt per min

EXAMPLE #3: Administer 500 mL of a 5% solution of normal serum albumin over 30 min. The drop factor is 10.

The Standard Formula

$$\frac{\text{Total volume} \times \text{Drop factor}}{\text{Total time (min)}} = \text{gtt/min}$$

$$\frac{500 \text{ mL} \times 10 \text{ gtt/mL}}{30 \text{ min}} = \frac{5,000}{30}$$

$$= 166.6 \text{ gtt/min}$$

ANSWER: 167 gtt per min

Dimensional Analysis

$$\frac{\text{Total volume}}{\text{hr}} = \frac{\text{Drop factor}}{\text{mL}} = \frac{1 \text{ hr}}{60 \text{ min}}$$

$$\frac{500 \text{ mL}}{0.5 \text{ hr}} \times \frac{10 \text{ gtt}}{1 \text{ mL}} \times \frac{1 \text{ hr}}{60 \text{ min}}$$

$$\frac{500 \times 10 \text{ (gtt)} \times 1}{0.5 \times 1 \times 60 \text{ (min)}} = \frac{5,000}{30}$$

$$= 166.6 \text{ gtt/min}$$

ANSWER: 167 gtt per min

Constant Factors

Quick Formula with Constant Factor

$$\frac{\text{Milliliters per hour (mL/hr)}}{\text{Constant factor}}$$
$$= \text{Drops per minute (gtt/min)}$$

The constant factor is derived from the drop factor (of the administration set) divided into the fixed time factor of 60 min. It can only be used with the time factor of 60 min. Because the drop factor of 60 has the same numerical value as 60 min, these numbers cancel themselves out. A constant factor of 1 can be used in the division to replace both of these numbers. Therefore, for this Quick Formula, you can use the constant factor (1) to replace 60 min and 60 gtt per mL.

Because 60 remains constant for this Quick Formula, you can calculate constant factors for other drop factors by dividing by 60. For example, when working with a drop factor of 10, you can use the constant factor of 6 (60 ÷ 10); 15 would give a constant factor of 4 (60 ÷ 15), and 20 would give a constant factor of 3 (60 ÷ 20).

EXAMPLE: Administer 1,000 mL of RL over 10 hr. The drop factor is 15 drops per mL.

Use the Quick Formula to Calculate mL per hr

CALCULATE
mL PER HR:
$$\frac{\text{Total volume}}{\text{Total hours}} = \text{Milliliters per hour}$$

$$\frac{1{,}000 \text{ mL}}{10 \text{ hr}} = 100 \text{ mL/hr}$$

Use the Constant Factor to Calculate Drops per Minute

$$\frac{\text{mL/hr}}{\text{Constant factor}} = \text{gtt/min}$$

$$\frac{100 \text{ mL/hr}}{4\,(60 \div 15)} = 25 \text{ gtt/min}$$

ANSWER: 25 gtt per min

Intermittent Intravenous Administration

Intravenous Piggyback Medications

An intermittent intravenous infusion is an intravenous preparation (usually electrolytes or antibiotics) that is "piggybacked" (IVPB) or connected to an existing IV line. The IVPB solution, usually 50 mL to 100 mL, is administered over 30 min to 60 min or less. The tubing for the secondary set will be shorter than the primary set and will have a drop factor of 60. It should be hung higher than the existing IV to allow the force of gravity to override the infusion of the primary IV. Remember: The greater the height, the greater is the pressure, and the faster is the rate of infusion! See Figure 10.3. If a piggyback medication is to be given at the same time as the primary infusion, the bag/bottle is hung at the same height and the setup is referred to as a *tandem setup*. Smaller quantities of solution (100 mL to 150 mL) and medications can be given via a burette chamber. These volume-controlled sets (Buretrol, Soluset, and Volutrol) are frequently used for pediatric doses (see Chapter 14).

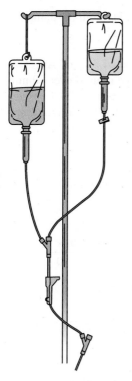

FIGURE 10.3 IV piggyback delivery system. (From Taylor, C., Lillis, C., and LeMone, P. [2001]. *Fundamentals of nursing. The art and science of nursing care* [4th ed.]. Philadelphia: Lippincott Williams & Wilkins.)

Frequently, the IVPB medication has to be reconstituted from a powder form (the type and amount of diluent will be specified), although some come premixed. You calculate the drip rate for the IVPB using the same formula that you used for the primary IV. If you are using an infusion pump, use the secondary IV setting and a drop factor of 60. Program the pump for the rate in mL per hr.

EXAMPLE: The physician ordered 1 g of Ancef in 100 mL of NS to be infused over 30 min via IVPB. The drop factor is 20 drops per mL. The IV should be infused at x drops per minute.

The Standard Formula

$$\frac{\text{Total volume} \times \text{Drop factor}}{\text{Time in minutes}}$$
$$= \text{Drops per minute}$$

$$\frac{100 \text{ mL} \times 20 \text{ (gtt/mL)}}{30 \text{ min}} = \frac{100 \times 20}{30}$$

$$= \frac{2{,}000}{30} = 66.6 \text{ gtt/min}$$

ANSWER: 67 gtt per min

Intravenous Push (IVP) Medications

Intravenous push medications should normally be given over 1 min to 5 min. Institution guidelines and reference materials provide acceptable rates of delivery and dilution requirements. Because the medication will have rapid effects, the total volume should be divided by the total minutes and then further divided into 15-sec increments. Use a watch to verify the time of infusion. See Figure 10.4.

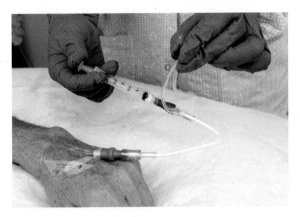

FIGURE 10.4 IV push medication. (From Taylor, C., Lillis, C., LeMone, P., and Lynn, P. [2008]. *Fundamentals of nursing. The art and science of nursing care* [6th ed.]. Philadelphia: Lippincott Williams & Wilkins.)

EXAMPLE: The physician ordered 30 mL, IV push, STAT. The literature recommends dilution with 10 mL of NS and injection over 5 min. Flush with 10 mL of NS.

Determine the total volume to be infused.
30 mL + 10 mL of dilution = 40 mL

$$\text{Use: } \frac{\text{Total volume}}{\text{Total minutes}}$$
$$= \text{Milliliters per minute}$$

$$\frac{40 \text{ mL}}{5 \text{ min}} = 8 \text{ mL/min}$$

Calculate mL to be given over 15 sec

Use: $\dfrac{\text{Total volume}}{4\ (60 \div 15\ \text{sec})}$

Milliliters over 15 sec

$\dfrac{8\ \text{mL}}{4} = 2\ \text{mL every 15 sec}$

ANSWER: 2 mL given every 15 sec
Flush with 10 mL of NS

PRACTICE PROBLEMS

1. The physician prescribed 1,000 mL of RL to infuse over 12 hr. You should give _____ mL per hr.

Critical Thinking Check

Does it seem logical that if 1,000 mL is to be infused over 12 hr, the hourly amount would be <100 mL? _____ **Yes or No?**

2. You are to give 500 mL of NS over 4 hr. You should give _____ mL per hr.

3. Administer 800 mL of NS over 10 hr. The drop factor is 20 drops per mL. You should give _____ drops per min.

4. You are to give 1,000 mL of 0.45% NS to infuse over 6 hours. The drop factor is 15 drops per mL. You should give _____ drops per min.

5. Administer 500 mL of solution over 24 hr. The drop factor is 60 drops per mL. You should give _____ drops per min.

6. You are to give 600 mL of solution over 12 hr. The drop factor is 20 drops per mL. You should give _____ drops per min.

> ### Critical Thinking Check
>
> Should you expect the rate of the infusion to be faster or slower if the drop factor was 15 gtt per mL instead of 20 gtt per mL? _____ **Faster or slower?**

7. The physician prescribed an IV of 100 mL of D5W to run at 100 mL per hr. The drop factor is 10. You should set the flow rate at _____ drops per min.

8. The physician prescribed an IV of 500 mL of Ringer's lactate at 75 mL per hr. The drop factor is 15. You should administer _____ drops per min.

9. The physician prescribed an IV of 250 mL of NS to be run at 50 mL per hr. The drop factor is 20. You should run the IV at _____ drops per min.

10. Give 50 mg of an antibiotic in 100 mL of D5W over 30 min. The drop factor is 15 drops per mL. You should piggyback this medication into the main IV and give at _____ drops per min.

11. The physician prescribed an IV of 1,500 mL of Ringer's lactate solution to infuse over 20 hr. The drop factor is 15 gtt per mL. You should give _____ drops per min.

12. Administer 1 g of an antibiotic in 50 mL of D5W over 30 min. The drop factor is 10 gtt per mL. The nurse should give _____ drops per min.

13. The physician prescribed an IV of 250 mL of D5 0.22% NS to infuse over 10 hr. The drop factor is 60 drops per min. The nurse should give _____ mL per hr and _____ drops per min.

> ### Critical Thinking Check
> If the drop factor of 60 is equal to the number of minutes in an hour (60), does it seem logical that the gtt per min should always equal the mL per hr? _____ **Yes or No?**

14. Administer 1 g of an antibiotic in 100 mL of D5W to run over 30 min. The drop factor is 20 drops per mL. You should give _____ drops per min.

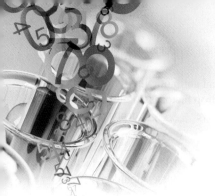

Complete the following IV calculations:

1. To infuse 500 mL of solution over 8 hr, you should give _____ mL per hr.

2. Administer 1,000 mL over 10 hr. You should give _____ mL per hr.

3. To deliver 1,000 mL of D5 0.45% NS over 4 hr, the nurse should administer _____ mL per hr.

4. To deliver 500 mL of D5W over a 6-hr period, the nurse should set the flow rate to deliver _____ mL per hr.

5. To deliver 250 mL of NS over a 5-hr period, the nurse should set the flow rate to deliver _____ mL per hr.

6. A patient is to receive 500 mL of 0.45% NS to run over 8 hr. The drop factor is 20 drops per mL. The nurse should give _____ mL per hr.

7. Administer 1,000 mL of 0.9% NS over 8 hr. The drop factor is 10 drops per mL. The flow rate should be _____ drops per min.

8. Administer 500 mL of D5W over a 12-hr period as KVO. The microdrip provides 60 drops per mL. Use the Quick Formula with the constant factor. The flow rate should be _____ drops per min.

9. To administer 1.0 L of Ringer's lactate over 6 hr, you should give _____ mL per hr. The drop factor is 10 drops per mL. The flow rate should be _____ drops per min.

10. The physician prescribed 1,000 mL of D5W to infuse over 24 hr. With a drop factor of 15 drops per mL, you should give _____ drops per min. Use the Quick Formula with the constant factor.

11. The physician prescribed 1,000 mL of D5W 0.9% NS to infuse at 75 mL per hr. The drop factor is 15 drops per mL. You should give _____ drops per min.

12. Ringer's lactate, 500 mL, is to infuse at 50 mL per hr. The drop factor is 10. You should set the rate at _____ drops per min. Use the Quick Formula and the constant factor.

13. Administer 1,000 mL of RL at 50 mL per hr. The total infusion time should be _____ hr.

14. You are to give 500 mL of NS at 40 mL per hr. The total infusion time should be _____ hr.

15. The physician prescribed 250 mL of D5W at 20 mL per hr. The total infusion time should be _____ hr.

16. The physician prescribed 100 mL of albumin to be absorbed over 2 hr. The drop factor is 15 drops per mL. The nurse should run the IV at _____ drops per min.

17. A patient is to receive 1,000 mL of NS with 20,000 units of heparin over 24 hr. The drop factor is 60 drops per mL. The nurse should give _____ drops per min.

18. A patient is to receive 350 mg of an antibiotic in 150 mL of D5W over a 1-hr period of time. The drop factor is 15 drops per mL. The nurse should give _____ drops per min.

19. Administer 100 mL of an antibiotic solution via an infusion pump over 60 min. The microdrip provides 60 drops per mL. You should give _____ drops per min.

20. The physician prescribed 500 mL of a 10% Intralipid solution to infuse over 4 hr. Using a pump, the nurse should set the rate at _____ mL per hr.

thePoint₂ Additional practice problems to enhance learning and facilitate chapter comprehension can be found on **http://thePoint.lww.com/Boyer8e.**

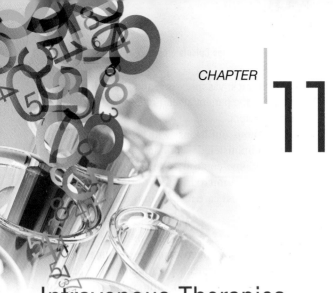

Intravenous Therapies
CRITICAL CARE APPLICATIONS

LEARNING OBJECTIVES

After completing this chapter, you should be able to:

- Calculate flow rate when critical care dosage is known.
- Calculate critical care dosages, per hour and per minute.
- Titrate IV fluids.

*I*n critical care situations small amounts of potent medications are ordered intravenously and must be carefully monitored. Some medications are ordered in units to be given over a specified time (e.g., heparin and insulin). Other medications are ordered by amount of drug. Frequently, the dosage is based on the patient's weight in kilograms. Some very potent medications (antiarrhythmics, vasopressors, and vasodilators) may be titrated to the patient's heart rate, blood pressure, or other parameters.

Intravenous infusions with critical care drugs must be administered with an electronic infusion pump or volume-controlled device. If these are not available, then a microdrip set at 60 drops per mL is necessary. Critical care medications can be prescribed accordingly:

- grams per minute (g per min), milligrams per minute (mg per min), micrograms per minute (mcg per min), or milliequivalents per minute (mEq per min)
- grams per hour (g per hr), milligrams per hour (mg per hr), micrograms per hour (mcg per hr), or milliequivalents per hour (mEq per hr)
- grams per kilogram per minute (g/kg/min), milligrams per kilogram per minute (mg/kg/min), micrograms per kilogram per minute (mcg/kg/min), or milliequivalents per kilogram per minute (mEq/kg/min).

The nurse must be able to calculate both the desired dosage and mL per hr for the IV infusion. *Remember:* You must always know the safe dosage dilution and rate of the medications you are administering before you begin the infusion. Refer to institutional guidelines or drug references when necessary.

This chapter will focus on critical care problems. Heparin and insulin infusions will be covered in their respective chapters. Refer to Appendix J for a review of nursing considerations for critical care drug administration. Please note: Due to the size of this book, only a small sampling of critical care problems can be provided here.

thePoint: Additional practice problems to enhance learning and facilitate chapter comprehension can be found on **http://thePoint.lww.com/Boyer8e.**

Calculate Flow Rate (mL per hr) When Dosage Is Known. Use Ratio and Proportion, the Formula Method, or Dimensional Analysis

To calculate milliliters per hour, you use one of the same three methods shown in Chapter 10. Note: When calculating critical care infusions, do not round up to the whole number if the pump can be set in tenths. The rate is more likely to be changed to a whole number when the dosage is titrated and then the dosage change is documented.

RULE

To calculate flow rate (mL per hr) when the dosage is known: Convert to like units, calculate dosage per kilogram per minute or per kilogram per hour if the drug is ordered by weight, change dosage per minute to dosage per hour (multiply by 60 before or after you calculate mL per hr), if dosage is ordered per minute, and calculate mL per hr using ratio and proportion, the Formula Method, or dimensional analysis.

EXAMPLE #1: Give a critical care medication, 500 mg in 250 mL D5W, at 5 mcg/kg/min for a patient weighing 152 lb. The electronic infusion pump should be set at _____ mL per hr.

CONVERT TO LIKE UNITS:
Change pounds to kilograms (2.2 lb = 1 kg): 152 lb ÷ 2.2 lb/kg = 69.1 or 69 kg.
Change milligrams to micrograms (1 mg = 1,000 mcg): 500 mg × 1,000 mcg/mg = 500,000 mcg

CALCULATE MCG/MIN:
5 mcg/kg/min × 69 kg = 345 mcg/min

Ratio and Proportion

345 mcg/min : x mL = 500,000 mcg : 250 mL
500,000x = 345 mcg/min × 250 mL
500,000x = 86,250

$$x = \frac{86,250}{500,000} = 0.1725 \text{ mL/min}$$

(carry out two spaces to hundredths)

CALCULATE ML/HR:
0.17 mL/min × 60 min/hr = 10.2 mL/hr

ANSWER: 10.2 mL per hr

The Formula Method

CALCULATE ML/MIN USING FORMULA:
$$\frac{D}{H} \times Q = x$$

$$\frac{345 \text{ mcg/min}}{500,000 \text{ mcg}} \times 250 \text{ mL}$$

$$x = \frac{86,250}{500,000} = 0.1725 \text{ mL/min}$$

(carry out two spaces to hundredths)

CALCULATE mL/HR: 0.17 mL/min × 60 min/hr = 10.2 mL/hr

ANSWER: 10.2 mL per hr

Dimensional Analysis

To set up this equation, you will need to use three conversion factors: 1 mg = 1,000 mcg; 60 min = 1 hr; and 1 kg = 2.2 lb.

$$\frac{5 \ \cancel{mcg}}{\cancel{kg/min}} \times \frac{250 \ (mL)}{500 \ \cancel{mg}} \times \frac{1 \ \cancel{mg}}{1,000 \ \cancel{mcg}}$$

$$\times \frac{60 \ \cancel{min}}{1 \ hr} \times \frac{1 \ \cancel{kg}}{2.2 \ \cancel{lb}} \times \frac{152 \ \cancel{lb}}{}$$

$$= \frac{5 \times 250 \ (mL) \times 1 \times 60 \times 1 \times 152}{500 \times 1,000 \times 1 \ (hr) \times 2.2}$$

$$= \frac{\cancel{11,400,000}^{114}}{\cancel{1,100,000}_{11}}$$

$$= \frac{114}{11} = 10.4 \ mL/hr \ or \ 10 \ mL/hr$$

ANSWER: 10.4 mL per hr

EXAMPLE #2: The physician ordered 400 mcg of Precedex in 100 mL of NS to infuse at 0.3 mcg/kg/hr for a person who weighs 132 lb.

CONVERT TO LIKE UNITS: Convert pounds to kilograms
132 lb ÷ 2.2 lb/kg = 60 kg

CALCULATE MCG/HR: 0.3 mcg/kg/hr × 60 kg = 18 mcg/hr

Ratio and Proportion

18 mcg/hr : x mL = 400 mcg : 100 mL
$400x$ = 18 mcg/hr × 100 mL
$400x$ = 1,800

$$x = \frac{1,800}{400} = 4.5 \text{ mL/hr}$$

ANSWER: 4.5 mL per hr

The Formula Method

$$\frac{D}{H} \times Q = x$$

$$\frac{18 \text{ mcg/hr}}{400 \text{ mcg}} \times 100 \text{ mL} = 4.5 \text{ mL/hr}$$

ANSWER: 4.5 mL per hr

Dimensional Analysis

To set up this equation, you will need one conversion factor: 1 kg = 2.2 lb.

$$\frac{0.3 \text{ meg}}{\text{kg}/\text{hr}} = \frac{100 \text{ (mL)}}{400 \text{ meg}}$$

$$= \frac{1 \text{ kg}}{2.2 \text{ lb}} = 132 \text{ lb}$$

$$\frac{0.3 \times 100 \text{ (mL)} \times 1 \times 132}{400 \times 2.2}$$

$$= \frac{3,960}{880} = 4.5 \text{ mL/hr}$$

ANSWER: 4.5 mL per hr

EXAMPLE #3: The physician ordered 900 mg of amiodarone in 500 mL D5W to run at 0.5 mg/min. How many milliliters per hour should the patient receive?

Ratio and Proportion

900 mg : 500 mL = 0.5 mg/min : x mL
$900x = 250 \; (= 500 \times 0.5)$

$$x = \frac{\cancel{250}^{\,25}}{\cancel{900}_{\,90}} = \frac{25}{90} = 0.277$$

(0.28) mL/min

CALCULATE ML/HR: 0.28 mL/min × 60 min/hr = 16.8 mL/hr

ANSWER: 16.8 mL per hr

The Formula Method

CALCULATE MG/MIN USING FORMULA:

$$\frac{D}{H} \times Q = x$$

$$\frac{0.5 \text{ mg/min}}{900 \text{ mg}} \times 500 \text{ mL}$$

$$= 0.278 \text{ mL/min } (0.28 \text{ mL/min})$$

CALCULATE ML/HR: 0.28 mL/min × 60 min/hr
= 16.8 mL/hr

ANSWER: 16.8 mL per hr

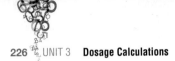

Dimensional Analysis

To set up this equation, you will only need one conversion factor: 60 min = 1 hr.

$$\frac{0.5 \text{ mg}}{\text{minute}} \times \frac{500 \text{ mL}}{900 \text{ mg}} \times \frac{60 \text{ min}}{1 \text{ hr}}$$

$$= \frac{0.5 \times 500 \text{ (mL)} \times 60}{900 \times 1 \text{ (hr)}} = \frac{\overset{150}{15,000}}{\underset{9}{900}}$$

$$= \frac{150}{9} = 16.7 \text{ mL/hr}$$

ANSWER: 16.7 mL per hr

Calculate Dosage, per Hour or per Minute, When Flow Rate Is Known

_R U L E_

To calculate dosage when the flow rate (mL per hr) is known: Convert to like units and calculate the dose (grams per minute, milligrams per minute, micrograms per minute) using ratio and proportion, the Formula Method, or dimensional analysis. If the drug is ordered by weight, calculate dosage per kilogram per minute (g/kg/min, mg/kg/min, mcg/kg/min).

EXAMPLE #1: A medication, 400 mg in 250 mL D5W, is to be infused at 20 mL/hr to maintain a systolic blood pressure (BP) of 100 mm Hg in a patient weighing 110 lb. How many mcg/kg/min should be infusing?

Ratio and Proportion

CONVERT TO
LIKE UNITS:
Change mg to mcg (400 mg ×
1,000 mcg/mg = 400,000 mcg)
Convert pounds to kilograms
110 lb ÷ 2.2 lb/kg = 50 kg

CALCULATE
MCG/HR:
400,000 mcg : 250 mL = x : 20 mL/hr
250x = 8,000,000 (400,000 × 20)

$$x = \frac{8,000,000}{250} = 32,000 \text{ mcg/hr}$$

CHANGE MCG/
HR TO MCG/MIN:
32,000 mcg/hr ÷ 60 min = 533 mcg/min

CHANGE TO
MCG/KG/MIN:
533 mcg/min ÷ 50 kg = 10.66 mcg/kg/
min

ANSWER: 10.7 mcg/kg/min

The Formula Method

CONVERT TO
LIKE UNITS:
Change mg to mcg (400 mg × 1,000
mcg/mg = 400,000 mcg)
Convert pounds to kilograms
110 lb ÷ 2.2 lb/kg = 50 kg

CONVERT mL/
HR TO mL/MIN:
20 mL/hr ÷ 60 min = 1,200 mL/min

USE
$\frac{D}{H} \times Q = x$

$$\frac{x \text{ mcg/min}}{400,000 \text{ mcg}} \times 250 \text{ mL}$$
$$= 0.33 \text{ mL/min}$$
$$0.000625x = 0.33$$
$$x = 528 \text{ mL/min}$$

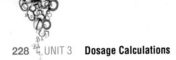

CHANGE TO MCG/KG/MIN:	528 mcg/min ÷ 50 kg = 10.56 mcg/kg/min (10.6)

ANSWER: 10.6 mcg/kg/min

Dimensional Analysis

To set up this equation, you will use three conversion factors (1 mg = 1,000 mcg, 60 min = 1 hr, and 2.2 lb = 1 kg) to get mcg/kg/minute.

- Use three conversion factors

$$\frac{20 \ \cancel{mL}}{1 \ \cancel{hr}} = \frac{400 \ \cancel{mg}}{250 \ \cancel{mL}} = \frac{1{,}000 \ (mcg)}{1 \ \cancel{mg}}$$

$$= \frac{1 \ \cancel{hr}}{60 \ min} \ \frac{2.2 \ \cancel{lb}}{1 \ kg} 110 \ lb$$

$$\frac{20 \times 400 \times 1{,}000 \ (mcg) \times 1 \times 2.2}{1 \times 250 \times 1 \times 60 \times 1 \times 110}$$

$$= \frac{17{,}600{,}000}{1{,}650{,}000}$$

$$= 10.66 \ (10.7) \ mcg/kg/min$$

ANSWER: 10.7 mcg/kg/min

EXAMPLE #2:	A physician prescribes 4 mg of a drug in 250 mL D5W to be titrated to 4 mL per hr to control pain in a patient who weighs 115 lb. How many mcg/kg/hr or mcg/kg/min should be infused?

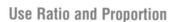

Use Ratio and Proportion

CONVERT TO LIKE UNITS: Change mg to mcg (4 mg × 1,000 mcg/mg = 4,000 mcg)
Change 115 lb to kg (115 lbs ÷ 2.2 lb/kg = 52 kg)

CALCULATE MCG/HR: 4,000 mcg : 250 mL = x : 4 mL/hr
$250x = 16,000$ (4,000 × 4)

$$x = \frac{16,000}{250} = 64 \text{ mcg/hr}$$

CALCULATE DOSAGE IN MCG/KG/HR: 64 mcg/hr ÷ 52 kg = 1.23 mcg/kg/hr

CHANGE TO MCG/KG/MIN: 1.23 mcg/kg/min ÷ 60 min = 0.02 mcg/kg/min

ANSWER: 1.23 mcg/kg/hr
or 0.02 mcg/kg/min

The Formula Method

CONVERT TO LIKE UNITS: Change mg to mcg (4 mg × 1,000 mcg/mg = 4,000 mcg)
Change 115 lb to kg (115 lb ÷ 2.2 lb/kg = 52 kg)

CALCULATE MCG/HR:
$$\frac{D}{H} \times Q = x$$

$$\frac{x \text{ mcg/hr}}{4,000 \text{ mcg}} \times 250 \text{ mL} = 4 \text{ mL/hr}$$

$0.0625x = 4$ mL/hr
$x = 64$ mcg/hr

CALCULATE
DOSAGE IN
MCG/KG/HR:

$$64 \text{ mcg} \div 52 \text{ kg} = 1.23 \text{ mcg/kg/hr}$$

CHANGE TO
MCG/KG/MIN:

$$1.23 \text{ mcg/kg/hr} \div 60 \text{ min} = 0.02 \text{ mcg/kg/min}$$

ANSWER: 1.23 mcg/kg/hr
or 0.02 mcg/kg/min

Dimensional Analysis

To set up this equation, you will need to use two conversion factors (1 mg = 1,000 mcg and 1 kg = 2.2 lb) to get mcg/kg/hr and three conversion factors (1 mg = 1,000 mcg; 60 min = 1 hr; and 1 kg = 2.2 lb) to get mcg/kg/min.

- Use two conversion factors

$$\frac{4 \text{ mL}}{\text{hour}} = \frac{4 \text{ mg}}{250 \text{ mL}} = \frac{1,000 \text{ mcg}}{1 \text{ mg}}$$

$$= \frac{2.2 \text{ lb}}{1 \text{ kg}} = 115 \text{ lb}$$

$$\frac{4 \times 4 \times 1,000 \text{ (mcg)} \times 1 \times 2.2}{1 \times 250 \times 1 \times 115}$$

$$= \frac{35,200}{28,750} = 1.22 \text{ mcg/kg/hr}$$

- Use three conversion factors

$$\frac{4 \text{ mL}}{\text{hour}} = \frac{4 \text{ mg}}{250 \text{ mL}} = \frac{1,000 \text{ mcg}}{1 \text{ mg}}$$

$$= \frac{1 \text{ hr}}{60 \text{ min}} = \frac{2.2 \text{ lb}}{1 \text{ kg}} = 115 \text{ lb}$$

$$\frac{4 \times 4 \times 1,000 \ (mcg) \times 1 \times 1 \times 2.2}{250 \times 1 \times 60 \times 1 \times 115}$$

$$= \frac{35,200}{1,725,000} = 0.02 \ mcg/kg/hr$$

ANSWER: 1.22 mcg/kg/hr
or 0.02 mcg/kg/min

Titrate IV Fluids

When a medication is titrated (e.g., dopamine, Neo-Synephrine), the lowest dose of medication is given first, and then the dosage is increased or decreased to achieve the desired result. Sometimes a bolus dose is initially given. An infusion pump should always be used, so you will need to calculate the infusion in mL per hr.

RULE

When solving a solution problem involving titration:
- Convert to like units.
- Calculate the concentration in mcg per mL.
- Convert the upper and lower dose ranges into mL/min.
- Convert mL per min into mL per hr.

EXAMPLE: A critical care medication was ordered to be titrated (2 to 4 mcg per min) to maintain a systolic blood pressure below 130 mm Hg. The solution being titrated contains 25 mg of medication in 500 mL D5W. The nurse needs to determine the setting for the infusion pump. The nurse should set the pump to x mL per hr.

| **CONVERT TO LIKE UNITS:** | 25 mg = 25,000 mcg (1 mg = 1,000 mcg) |

CONVERT THE UPPER AND LOWER DOSE RANGES INTO mL/MIN:

The solution concentration is 50 mcg/mL
25,000 mcg : 500 mL = 2 mcg/min : x
$25,000x = 1,000$ (= 2 × 500)

$$x = \frac{1,000}{25,000} = \frac{1}{25} = 0.04$$

$x = 0.04$ mL/min = *lower dosage range*
25,000 mcg : 500 mL = 4 mcg : x
$25,000x = 2,000$ (= 4 × 500)

$$x = \frac{2,000}{25,000} = \frac{2}{25} = \frac{1}{12.5} = 0.08$$

$x = 0.08$ mL/min = *upper dosage range*

CONVERT mL/ MIN TO mL/HR:

Lower dosage range: 0.04 × 60 min = 2.4 mL/hr
Upper dosage range: 0.08 × 60 min = 4.8 mL/hr

ANSWER: The nurse should titrate the dosage range of 2 to 4 mcg per min by setting the pump to infuse at a flow rate of 2.4 to 4.8 mL per hr.

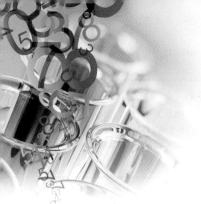

Complete the following problems:

1. The physician prescribes 50 mg of a drug in
   250 mL D5W to start at 10 mcg per min to
   relieve chest pain. You should set the infusion
   pump at _____ mL per hr.

> ### Critical Thinking Check
>
> If the prescribed dosage is doubled to 20 mcg
> per min, would you expect the infusion pump
> setting to double (set at 6 mL per hr)? _____
> **Yes or No?**

2. The nurse increased a lidocaine infusion of 2 g
   in 250 mL D5W to 30 mL per hr to control the
   patient's dysrhythmia. You should document that
   the patient is now receiving _____ mg per min.

3. The physician prescribes dopamine 400 mg in
   250 mL D5W to start at 5 mcg/kg/min for a
   patient weighing 178 lb. You should set the
   infusion pump at _____ mL per hr.

Critical Thinking Check

If the physician prescribed 800 mg of dopamine in 250 mL at 5 mcg/kg/min, would you expect the mL per hr to _____ **Increase, Decrease, or Remain the Same?**

---

4. A 75-kg patient on a mechanical ventilator is sedated with propofol (Diprivan) 1,000 mg in 100 mL at 10 mL per hr. You should document that the patient is receiving _____ mcg/kg/min.

5. The physician prescribes lorazepam (Ativan) 250 mg in 250 mL to run at 3 mg per hr. You should set the infusion pump at _____ mL per hr.

6. The physician prescribes a continuous infusion of a drug to control hypertension. The label directs you to remove 90 mL from a 250-mL NS bag and add 200 mg of the medication. The medication vial has 5 mg per mL. You should add _____ mL of the drug to the IV bag. The concentration of medication should be _____ mg per mL (remember to include the volume of the of the drug in the calculation of the total volume). In order to administer 1 mg per min, you should set the infusion pump at _____ mL per hr.

7. The physician prescribes a loading dose of procainamide 500 mg in 100 mL NS over 30 min. The label reads procainamide 500 mg per mL. You should add _____ mL of procainamide to 100 mL NS. You should set the infusion pump at

_____ mL per hr to deliver this bolus. The load-
ing dose is to be followed with a continuous
infusion of procainamide 2 g in 250 mL D5W to
run at 2 mg per min. You should set the infusion
pump at _____ mL per hr.

8. A patient is to receive a diltiazem (Cardizem)
   bolus of 10 mg followed by a continuous infusion of Cardizem at 10 mg per hr. The Cardizem
   vials contain 5 mg per mL. To administer the
   bolus you should give _____ mL over 2 min. To
   mix the continuous infusion you should inject
   125 mg in a 100-mL bag of NS. You should add
   _____ mL of Cardizem to the IV bag. Keeping
   in mind the new total volume in the IV bag, you
   should set the infusion pump at _____ mL per hr
   to deliver 10 mg per hr.

9. Dopamine 800 mg in 250 mL D5W is infusing at
   12 mL per hr in a patient weighing 195 lb. You
   should document that the patient is receiving
   _____ mcg/kg/min.

C r i t i c a l   T h i n k i n g   C h e c k

If the flow rate were to increase to 18 mL per hr,
would you expect the mcg/kg/min to _____
Increase or Decrease?

---

10. The physician prescribes phenylephrine (Neo-
    Synephrine) 100 mg in 250 mL D5W continuous
    infusion to run at 50 mcg per min. You should set
    the infusion pump at _____ mL per hr.

To maintain the systolic BP above 90 mm Hg, the rate is increased to 12 mL per hr. You document that the patient is now receiving _____ mcg per min.

11. Tirofiban (Aggrastat) 12.5 mg in 250 mL is prescribed to be infused at a rate of 0.1 mcg/kg/min in a patient weighing 82 kg. You should set the pump at _____ mL per hr.

12. A hypertensive patient weighs 165 lb. His physician prescribed nitroprusside (Nipride) 3 mcg/kg/min, IV. Nipride 50 mg is added to a 250-mL solution of D5W. This solution should contain a concentration of Nipride, _____ mcg per mL. Using an infusion pump, the nurse should set the flow rate at _____ mL per hr.

13. A patient is to receive nitroglycerine (Nitrostat) 20 mcg per min, IV. Nitrostat is available in a 10-mL vial labeled 5 mg per mL. To prepare a 200-mcg per mL solution, with a concentration of 50 mg in 250 mL, the nurse should add _____ mL of Nitrostat to 250 mL of D5W and set the infusion pump flow rate at _____ mL per hr to deliver 20 mcg per min.

14. Give 400 mg of dopamine in 250 mL of D5NS to infuse at 300 mcg per min. Calculate flow rate in mL per hr. You should give _____ mL per hr.

Critical Thinking Check

If the infusion increased to 500 mcg per min, should you expect the mL per hr to _____ **Increase or Decrease?** If the quantity of solution increased to 500 mL of D5NS, at the same infusion of 300 mcg per min, should the mL per hr _____ **Increase or Decrease?**

---

15. A patient is started on a furosemide (Lasix) infusion to promote diuresis. Lasix 2,000 mg in 200 mL is prescribed at 1 mg per min. You should set the pump at _____ mL per hr.

16. A patient is started on norepinephrine 4 mg in 250 mL D5W at 15 mL per hr. You should document that the patient is receiving _____ mcg per min.

17. Octreotide (Sandostatin) 1,250 mcg in 250 mL is prescribed at 50 mcg per hr. Using an infusion pump, you should set the rate at _____ mL per hr.

18. A patient is to receive dobutamine 1,000 mg in 250 mL NS at 10 mcg/kg/min to maintain a systolic BP of 90 mm Hg. In a patient weighing 95 kg, you should set the pump at _____ mL per hr.

thePoint. Additional practice problems to enhance learning and facilitate chapter comprehension can be found on **http://thePoint.lww.com/Boyer8e.**

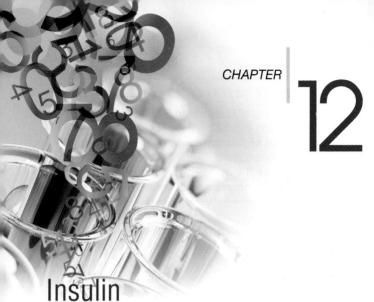

12

Insulin

LEARNING OBJECTIVES

After completing this chapter, you should be able to:

- Explain the purpose of insulin.
- List the different types of insulin.
- Compare the four different types of insulin preparations (rapid acting, short acting, intermediate acting, and long acting) according to onset, peak, and duration.
- Distinguish between a standard 1-mL (100-unit) syringe and a 0.5-mL (50-unit) syringe.
- Distinguish among the various types of insulin devices.
- Explain the concept of the sliding scale for insulin coverage.
- Describe the steps necessary to prepare insulin for injection.
- Describe the steps necessary to mix two types of insulin in one syringe.
- Describe how to use an insulin pump.

238

Insulin Preparation

Insulin is a natural hormone secreted by the islets of Langerhans in the pancreas to maintain blood sugar levels. Insulin enables the body to use glucose as a source of energy. When insulin is insufficient, blood sugar rises and insulin injections may be necessary.

The major insulin preparations in use today are the synthetic human insulins (Regular and NPH) and their analogs: aspart, glulisine, lispro (rapid acting), Levemir, and Lantus (long acting). Lente and Ultralente are being phased out.

All analog insulins are clear and colorless. Insulins are identified by trade and generic names. The insulin label identifies the source as "rDNA origin." The capitalized trade name (e.g., Humulin) on the insulin drug label is followed by a letter that indicates the type of insulin. The letter N refers to NPH (intermediate acting), and R refers to Regular (short acting). See Figures 12.1 and 12.2.

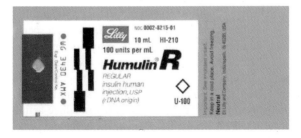

FIGURE 12.1 Humulin R. (Courtesy of Eli Lilly Company, Indianapolis, IN.)

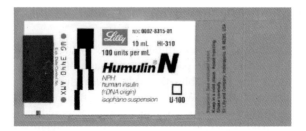

FIGURE 12.2 Humulin N. (Courtesy of Eli Lilly Company, Indianapolis, IN.)

Types of Insulin

Insulin is measured in units and supplied in 10-mL vials providing 100 units of insulin per milliliter. The most common insulin concentration is U-100. Insulin is also available as U-500 (500 units per milliliter) for individuals with difficult-to-manage blood sugar levels. This is a special order, and the vial of insulin should not be kept with the U-100 vials. A U-100 syringe is used for U-100 and should only be used *with extreme caution* (special order) for U-500 insulin.

Insulin is classified according to its onset, peak, and duration of action (rapid-acting, short-acting, intermediate-acting, and long-acting insulin). Rapid-acting insulin (lispro) is used when an effect is needed in 5 min to 30 min. Short-acting insulin (Regular) starts to work in 30 min to 60 min. Intermediate-acting insulin (NPH) usually takes 1½ hr for onset and peaks in 12 hr. Long-acting insulin (Lantus) can last for 24 hr and is used for once-daily dosing. Regular, aspart, and glulisine have been approved for IV use. See Table 12.1.

Table 12.1 **Insulin Type, Onset, Peak, and Duration of Action**

Insulin	Onset	Peak	Duration
Rapid-acting			
Apidra (glulisine)*	10–15 min	1/2–1 1/2 hr	3 hr or less
Humalog (lispro)	5 min	1 hr	2–4 hr
Novolog (aspart)*	10–20 min	1–3 hr	3–5 hr
Short-acting			
Humulin R (Regular)*	1/2–1 hr	2–3 hr	5–8 hr
Novolin R (Regular)	1/2 hr	2 1/2–5 hr	8 hr
ReliOn R (Novolin R)	1/2 hr	2 1/2–5 hr	8 hr
Intermediate-acting			
Humulin N (NPH)	1–3 hr	2–8 hr	14–24 hr
Novolin N (NPH)	1 1/2 hr	4–12 hr	24 hr
ReliOn N (Novolin N)	1 1/2 hr	4–12 hr	24 hr
Long-acting			
Lantus (insulin glargine)	1 hr	No	20–24 hr
Levemir (insulin detemir)	1–2 hr	No	Up to 24 hr

*Approved for IV use.

Insulin also comes in premixed combinations. The ratio of the combined insulin always equals 100%—for example, Novolin 70/30 (70% NPH and 30% Regular). Therefore, if a physician orders 30 units of Novolin 70/30, the 30 units that you draw from the vial would contain 21 units of NPH (70% of 30) and 9 units of Regular (30% of 30). Examples of other preparations are: Humalog 75/25, Humalog 50/50, NovoLog 70/30, Humulin 70/30, and Humulin 50/50. Note that N insulin does not indicate NovoLog insulin or Novolin 70/30. If a physician orders 25 units of N insulin, use only Humulin N (NPH), Novolin N (NPH), or ReliOn N. If Novolog or Novolin 70/30 were desired, then the full drug name would appear on the order.

Insulin Delivery Devices

There are a variety of insulin delivery devices: syringes; pens and pumps; and injection ports (Insulfon and the i-port). The size of this handbook prevents a comprehensive review of all devices. Therefore only a brief description of each will be provided.

Syringes

Insulin, which is always ordered and supplied in units, is given with a special 1-mL syringe *marked in units (100 units per milliliters)*. This syringe is only used for insulin! The most common, single-scale 1-mL (U-100) syringe is calibrated every 2 units, with every 10th unit marked in large numbers on one side (Figure 12.3 A). A double-scale 1-mL (U-100) syringe

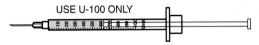

USE U-100 ONLY

A: Standard U-100 insulin syringe with 2-unit calibration markings every 10 units. *Shaded area* indicates 60 units of Regular insulin in a 1-mL syringe.

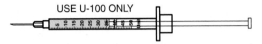

USE U-100 ONLY

B: A Lo-Dose U-50 insulin syringe with 1-unit calibration markings every 5 units. *Shaded area* indicates 35 units of Regular insulin in a 0.5-mL syringe.

FIGURE 12.3 Two common types of insulin syringes.

has 2-unit calibrations. Every 5 units are marked in large numbers on the left side, and every 10 units are marked on the right side. This makes it easier to accurately measure odd and even unit increments.

A 0.5-mL (Lo-Dose, Becton Dickinson) syringe is sized to hold no more than 50 units of U-100 insulin. Note that the insulin concentration is the same (100 units per milliliter), but the barrel of the syringe is thinner, reducing the syringe capacity to 0.5 mL (50 units). There are 1-unit calibration markings and large numbers every 5 units (Figure 12.3 B). The enlarged scale of the 0.5-mL syringe makes it easier to read. Patients are encouraged to choose the smallest syringe size that will contain the dose of insulin to be administered. The smaller 0.5-mL (holds up to 50 units of U-100 insulin) or 0.3-mL (holds up to 30 units of U-100 insulin) syringe is recommended sometimes for home use, but the 1-mL self-capping U-100 insulin syringes are preferred in medical facilities to reduce errors in dosing.

Pens and Pumps

Disposable Pens

Insulin is also available in prefilled, disposable pens or cartridges for reusable pens. Pens contain an insulin-filled cartridge. The reservoir should always be checked to make sure that the desired dose is available. A function check should be done prior to administering an insulin dose with a pen. Dial-in 1 to 2 units, and depress the button while holding the pen with the pen needle pointed upright. Watch for 1 or 2 drops of insulin to leave the pen needle to ensure proper pen function. Then dial-in the desired dose. The insulin is administered subcutaneously, using a darting technique. Make sure to fully depress the button on the pen. Hold the needle in the subcutaneous tissue to the count of 5 after administering the dose to ensure complete delivery. The pen needle is removed and discarded immediately after each use.

Insulin Pumps

Continuous subcutaneous insulin infusion pumps deliver a constant dose of rapid-acting insulin, at a preset (basal) rate of units per hour, via tubing and a plastic cannula or small needle inserted into the subcutaneous tissue. Multiple rates can be programmed. In addition, a specific dose (bolus) of rapid-acting insulin is programmed as needed to "cover" a meal or to "correct" for high glucose. Most insulin pumps in use today are individually programmed to calculate

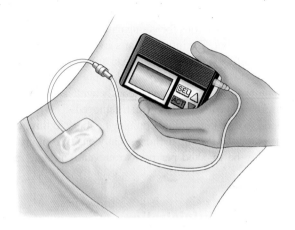

FIGURE 12.4 Insulin pump. (From Taylor, C., Lillis, C., LeMone, P., and Lynn, P. [2008]. *Fundamentals of nursing. The art and science of nursing care* [6th ed.]. Philadelphia: Lippincott Williams & Wilkins.)

"bolus" dosages based on the carbohydrate content of the meal and the current blood glucose level. The person using an insulin pump should insert a new infusion set in a new location every 48 hr to 72 hr. See Figure 12.4. Note that only short- or rapid-acting insulin is placed in the insulin pump reservoir! This insulin is drawn up from a conventional 10-mL vial of U-100 R or rapid analog insulin.

Spray Injectors, Injection Ports, Insulfon, and the i-port

The production of inhaled insulin has been suspended in the United States. Injection ports (Insulfon, i-port) are available and are sometimes used to reduce the number of injections for young children or adults with needle phobia. The infusion ports are similar to insulin pump infusion sets. Rather than tubing being connected to a constant insulin supply (pump), the cannula is inserted subcutaneously with a 31-gauge insertion needle, which is then removed. The port is taped to the skin, and insulin may be injected through the diaphragm for up to 3 days. Only one type of insulin may be injected per port to prevent "mixing" of insulins.

Insulin Administration

Insulin is never ordered orally or intramuscularly. A site rotation schedule is used to minimize the overuse of one area for subcutaneous injection. Insulin orders are written in units, and U-100 (100 units per milliliter) strength is used almost exclusively. Orders must include the type of insulin (e.g., Regular, Lantus), the units, the route (subcutaneous or IV), and the time (e.g., 1/2 hr before meals; at bedtime).

Sliding Scale Coverage

Sometimes patients receive additional rapid insulin during the day to correct high blood sugar. The dosage and frequency of insulin depend on the blood sugar level and are ordered using a sliding scale. Regular and rapid analog insulins (Novolog [aspart], Humalog [lispro], Apidra [glulisine]) are used. See Table 12.2.

Table 12.2   **Sample Sliding Scale for Insulin Coverage**

Blood Sugar (mg/dL)	Insulin Coverage
≤180	None
181–260	3 units
261–310	6 units
311–420	8 units
>421	10 units, call MD

Preparing Insulin for Injection

To prepare insulin for injection, follow these steps:

- Read the medication order, noting the type of insulin and number of units ordered. For example, a patient is ordered 60 units of NPH insulin.
- Select the correct insulin vial. Check the vial label three times. You should choose the vial of insulin marked N (Humulin N, Novolin N) 100 units per milliliter.
- Choose an insulin syringe large enough to hold 60 units. You should choose a 1-mL U-100 insulin syringe.
- Draw up the required dose by filling the syringe to the desired calibration. You would fill a 1-mL insulin syringe to the 60-unit line. Remember these tips:

  - Never shake the insulin vial! Always mix the suspended (cloudy) insulins by rolling between the palms of your hands. Regular insulin may be mixed in a syringe with NPH.

- The insulin analogs must never be mixed in a syringe with another insulin. Only R (short-acting) insulin or rapid-acting insulin analogs may be added to an IV.
- Refer to Appendix E for information about a sub-cutaneous injection.

Mixing Two Types of Insulin in One Syringe

Occasionally you will find it necessary to mix two types of insulin, usually Regular and NPH. Remember, Levemir and Lantus should never be mixed in a syringe with another insulin! When you have to mix insulins, there are *five important guidelines that you must remember:*

1. Do not contaminate the contents of one vial with the contents of the other vial.
2. Always draw up *Regular insulin first.*
3. Always *draw up the NPH insulin last* because chemically it has a protein substance in it that Regular insulin does not have. Drawing up the NPH insulin last helps prevent contamination of the Regular insulin.
4. Choose a 0.5-mL (50-unit) insulin syringe to measure smaller dosages; use a 1-mL (100-unit) insulin syringe for larger combinations.
5. Always add air into each vial equal to the amount of the required dose. Air prevents a vacuum from occurring. *Note:* Always inject air into the *NPH vial first!*

| EXAMPLE: | The physician prescribed 20 units of NPH and 10 units of Regular. To mix two types of insulin in one syringe for injection, Regular and NPH, follow these steps and refer to the illustrations A through G. |

- Check the medication order. Know the type of insulin ordered and the total number of units prescribed.
- Wash your hands and obtain the correct vials of U-100 NPH and Regular insulin and the correct U-100 syringe.
- Cleanse the tops of both vials with an alcohol swab. Regular is always clear and colorless in appearance. NPH is cloudy in appearance. Rotate the vial of NPH between the palms of your hands. *Never shake the vial*!
- Inject air equal to the insulin dose of NPH (20 units) into the NPH insulin vial first **(A)**. *Do not touch the insulin solution with the tip of the needle*. Remove the needle.
- Use the same syringe and inject air equal to the dose of Regular insulin (10 units) into the Regular insulin vial **(B)**. Be careful that the needle does not touch the solution because air should not be bubbled through the solution.

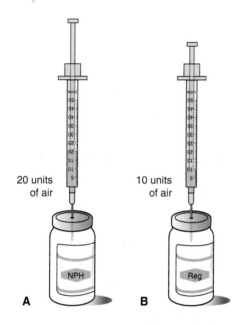

- Invert the vial of Regular insulin and draw back the required dosage (**C**). Check the dosage (10 units).
- Remove the syringe from the vial of Regular insulin (**D**) and check for air bubbles. Tap the syringe to remove any bubbles. If necessary, draw up additional medication for correct dosage.

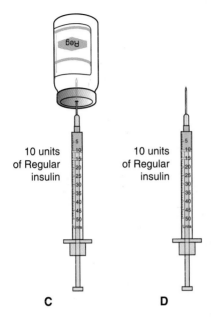

10 units
of Regular
insulin

C

10 units
of Regular
insulin

D

- Put the syringe into the NPH vial (**E**), being careful
  not to inject any Regular insulin into the NPH vial.
- Invert the vial of NPH and withdraw the required
  dosage (20 units) while holding the syringe at eye
  level. There should be a total of 30 units in the
  syringe (**F**).
- Check the dosage, which should be the addition of
  the two insulins (**G**). Air bubbles at this point indicate an incorrect dose, and the medication must be
  drawn up again.

• Prepare to administer the correct dose.

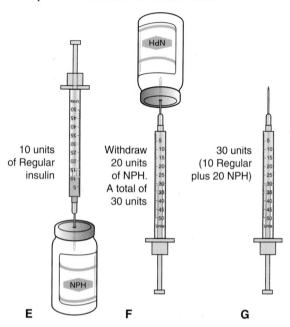

10 units
of Regular
insulin

Withdraw
20 units
of NPH.
A total of
30 units

30 units
(10 Regular
plus 20 NPH)

E   F   G

Continuous Intravenous Insulin Infusion

Administering insulin by continuous IV infusion requires using an infusion pump to guarantee accurate dosage and infusion rate. Consider the following.

EXAMPLE: The physician ordered 25 units of Regular insulin/hr, IV. Available is 125 units of Regular insulin in 250 mL NS. The infusion pump should be set to x mL/hr.

The Formula Method

$$\frac{D}{H} \times Q = x$$

$$\frac{25 \text{ units}}{125 \text{ units}} \times 250 \text{ mL}$$

$$\frac{\overset{1}{\cancel{25}}}{\underset{5}{\cancel{125}}} \times 250 = \frac{\overset{50}{\cancel{250}}}{\underset{1}{\cancel{5}}} = 50 \text{ mL}$$

ANSWER: Set the pump to deliver 50 mL/hr.

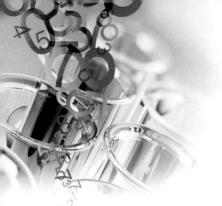

Complete the following problems:

Look at the following syringes and identify the correct dosage of insulin by using an arrow to mark your answer or shade in the areas.

1. Indicate 60 units U-100 insulin.

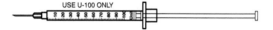

2. Indicate 82 units U-100 insulin.

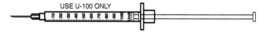

3. Indicate 45 units U-100 insulin.

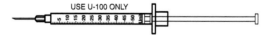

4. Indicate 35 units U-100 insulin.

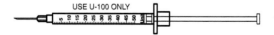

5. Indicate 10 units Regular U-100 insulin combined with 16 units NPH U-100 insulin.

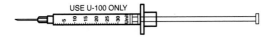

6. Indicate 16 units Regular U-100 insulin combined with 40 units NPH U-100 insulin.

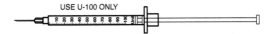

Identify the insulin dosage indicated by the shaded area on the following syringes.

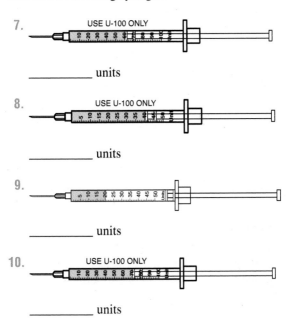

7.

_____ units

8.

_____ units

9.

_____ units

10.

_____ units

For the combined doses of insulin, indicate the total insulin dosage in the first column and the appropriate syringe (0.5 mL or 1 mL) in the second column.

	Total Dosage	Syringe/mL
11. 5 units Regular 16 units NPH	_____	_____
12. 30 units NPH 15 units Regular	_____	_____
13. 28 units Regular 36 units NPH	_____	_____
14. 18 units Regular 20 units NPH	_____	_____
15. 20 units NPH 10 units Regular	_____	_____

16. The physician ordered 30 units of U-100 Regular insulin to be given before lunch. You should select a _____ syringe and draw up _____ units of Regular insulin.

Critical Thinking Check

Does it seem logical or not logical to use a U-100 syringe because the Regular insulin is U-100? _____ **Logical or Not Logical?**

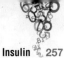

17. You have been asked to give 15 units of Humulin R insulin and 24 units of Humulin N. You should give a combined dose of _____ units in a _____ syringe.

18. The physician prescribed 15 units of Humulin R insulin to be given subcutaneously at 11:00 AM to cover a blood sugar reading of 325. The nurse should use a 0.5-mL syringe and draw up _____ units.

19. The physician prescribed 50 units of Humulin N insulin to be given subcutaneously at 8:00 AM. Using a 1-mL (100 unit) insulin syringe, the nurse should draw up _____ units.

Critical Thinking Check

There were only 1-mL syringes available for the 50-unit dose. Could the nurse have used a 0.5-mL syringe if it were available? _____ **Yes or No?**

---

20. The physician prescribed a combination of 22 units of NPH insulin and 12 units of Regular insulin. Using a U-50 insulin syringe, the nurse should draw up a total of _____ units, making certain to draw up the _____ insulin last.

thePoint· Additional practice problems to enhance learning and facilitate chapter comprehension can be found on **http://thePoint.lww.com/Boyer8e.**

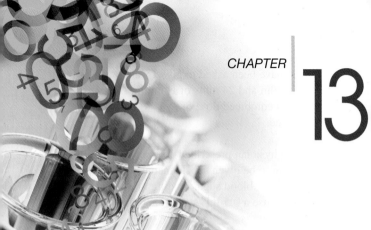

13

Heparin Preparation and Dosage Calculations
SUBCUTANEOUS AND INTRAVENOUS

LEARNING OBJECTIVES

After completing this chapter, you should be able to:

- Explain the purpose of heparin.
- Calculate heparin dosage for subcutaneous injection.
- Calculate heparin dosage for intravenous infusion.
- Calculate heparin flow rate (mL/hr) when heparin is ordered in units/hr.
- Calculate heparin dosage (units/hr) when heparin is ordered in mL/hr.
- Calculate heparin flow rate (mL/hr) when heparin is ordered based on weight (units/kg/hr).

- Explain the intravenous heparin protocol. Calculate bolus dose and infusion rate using an intravenous heparin protocol.

*H*eparin is an anticoagulant that prevents the formation of a new clot and the extension of an existing clot. Heparin is ordered in USP units (units/hr, units/kg/hr) or mL/hr. Heparin can be given subcutaneously or intravenously for intermittent (heparin lock) or continuous infusion using an electronic infusion pump.

Heparin is most effective when ordered based on weight (kg). The physician attempts to maintain a therapeutic anticoagulation level by titrating the dosage based on the laboratory results of the partial thromboplastin time (PTT). When heparin is prescribed based on weight, a bolus, or loading dose, is ordered in units/kg, followed by a continuous heparin infusion prescribed in units/kg/hr and given via an infusion pump. Lovenox is a commonly used low-molecular-weight anticoagulant ordered by weight (i.e., 1 mg per kg, twice daily) and administered subcutaneously. It is prepared in prefilled syringes in different amounts.

Heparin is available in single and multidose vials. Heparin is available in various solution strengths of units per mL: 10; 100; 1,000; 5,000; 10,000; 20,000; and 40,000. Saline flush solution (10 units per mL or 100 units per mL) is used periodically to maintain catheter patency. Central intravenous lines are flushed with 3 mL of a heparin lock solution (100 units per mL).

Subcutaneous heparin works in 20 min to 60 min, whereas IV heparin is immediate. The normal heparinizing adult dosage is 20,000 units to 40,000 units per 24 hr. See Figure 13.1.

To safely prepare heparin, first read the vial label carefully! Next, determine that the prescribed dose is within normal limits and can safely be given based on the patient's coagulation laboratory test results (PTT). Then, verify the route of administration and calculate the 24-hr dosage to estimate safety of drug administration.

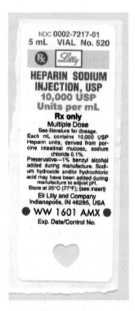

FIGURE 13.1 Heparin sodium injection. (Courtesy of Eli Lilly Company, Indianapolis, IN.)

Heparin for Subcutaneous Injection

_R U L E_

To prepare heparin for subcutaneous injection: Determine
that the dose is within the safe, normal range and calculate
the desired amount based on the available amount of the
dose. Use one of the three standard methods for dosage
calculation. Use a tuberculin or prepackaged syringe to
administer.

EXAMPLE #1:   Give heparin 5,000 units subcutaneously
every 6 hr.

CHECK: Determine if the prescribed dose is within
the normal heparinizing adult dosage for
24 hr. Heparin 5,000 units, q6h, equals
20,000 units in 24 hr (5,000 units
× 4 doses). This is within the safe normal
dosage.

SELECT: Select heparin 10,000 units per mL; 5-mL
vial.

Ratio and Proportion

10,000 units : 1 mL = 5,000 units : x mL
$10,000x = 5,000$

$$x = \frac{5,000^1}{10,000_2} = \frac{1}{2} = 0.5 \text{ mL}$$

ANSWER: 0.5 mL

The Formula Method

$$\frac{D}{H} \times Q = x$$

$$\frac{5,000 \text{ units}}{10,000 \text{ units}} \times 1 \text{ mL} = x$$

$$x = \frac{5,000^{1}}{10,000_{2}} = \frac{1}{2} = 0.5 \text{ mL}$$

ANSWER: 0.5 mL

Dimensional Analysis

$$5,000 \text{ units} \times \frac{1 \text{ (mL)}}{10,000 \text{ units}} =$$

$$= \frac{5,000 \times 1 \text{ (mL)}}{10,000 \text{ units}} = \frac{5,000 \text{ mL}}{10,000 \text{ units}}$$

$$= \frac{1}{2} = 0.5 \text{ mL}$$

ANSWER: 0.5 mL

EXAMPLE #2: A patient is prescribed 3,000 units of heparin to be administered subcutaneously every 12 hr.

CHECK: Determine if the prescribed dose is within the normal heparinizing adult dosage for 24 hours. Heparin 3,000 units, q12h, equals 6,000 units (= 3,000 × 2) in 24 hours. This is below the normal dosage and safe to give.

| SELECT: | Select heparin 5,000 units per mL; 10-mL vial. |

Ratio and Proportion

5,000 units : 1 mL = 3,000 units : x mL
$5,000x = 3,000$

$$x = \frac{3,000}{5,000}^{3}_{5} = \frac{3}{5} = 0.6 \text{ mL}$$

ANSWER: 0.6 mL

The Formula Method

$$\frac{D}{H} \times Q = x$$

$$\frac{3,000 \text{ units}}{5,000 \text{ units}} \times 1 \text{ mL} = x$$

$$\frac{3,000}{5,000}^{3}_{5} = \frac{3}{5} = 0.6 \text{ mL}$$

ANSWER: 0.6 mL

Dimensional Analysis

$$\frac{3,000 \text{ units}}{} \times \frac{1 \text{ mL}}{5,000 \text{ units}}$$

$$= \frac{3,000 \text{ units}}{} \times \frac{1 \text{ (mL)}}{5,000 \text{ units}}$$

$$= \frac{3,000 \times 1 \text{ (mL)}}{5,000} = \frac{3,000}{5,000}^{3}_{5} = \frac{3}{5} = 0.6$$

ANSWER: 0.6 mL

Heparin for Intravenous Infusion

Special calculations are required when administering IV heparin.

___RULE___

To add heparin to an IV: Calculate the desired quantity based on the available concentration. Use one of the three standard methods of calculation. The Formula Method will be used here as an example.

EXAMPLE: The physician ordered 25,000 units of heparin in 0.5 NS. Heparin is available in a vial marked 5,000 U/mL. How many mL of heparin should the nurse add to the IV fluid?

The Formula Method

$$\frac{D}{H} \times Q = x$$

$$\frac{25,000 \text{ units}}{5,000 \text{ units}} \times 1 \text{ mL} = x$$

$$\frac{25,000}{5,000} = \frac{25}{5} = \frac{5}{1} = 5 \text{ mL}$$

ANSWER: Add 5 mL of heparin to IV solution.

Calculate Heparin Flow Rate (mL/hr) When Units of Heparin per Hour Are Ordered

RULE

To calculate flow rate (mL per hr) when heparin is ordered in units per hour: Calculate the desired hourly amount based on the available amount. Use one of the three standard methods of calculation. Use an infusion pump to administer.

EXAMPLE #1:   The physician ordered 1,000 units per hr of heparin. You have available 500 mL of D5W with 20,000 units of heparin added. Calculate the flow rate in mL per hr.

Ratio and Proportion

20,000 units : 500 mL = 1,000 units : x mL
20,000x = 500,000 (500 × 1,000)

$$x = \frac{\cancel{500,000}^{\,25}}{\cancel{20,000}_{\,1}} = \frac{25}{1} = 25 \text{ mL/hr}$$

ANSWER: 25 mL per hr

The Formula Method

$$\frac{D}{H} \times Q = x$$

$$\frac{1,000 \text{ units}}{20,000 \text{ units}} \times 500 = x$$

$$\frac{\overset{1}{\cancel{1,000}} \text{ units}}{\underset{20}{\cancel{20,000}} \text{ units}} \times 500$$

$$\frac{1}{20} \times 500 = \frac{500}{20} = \frac{25}{1} = 25 \text{ mL/hr}$$

ANSWER: 25 mL per hr

Dimensional Analysis

$$\frac{1,000 \text{ units}}{\text{hr}} \times \frac{500 \text{ mL}}{20,000 \text{ units}}$$

$$\frac{1,000 \ \cancel{\text{units}}}{\text{hr}} \times \frac{500 \ (\text{mL})}{20,000 \ \cancel{\text{units}}}$$

$$= \frac{1,000 \times 500 \ (\text{mL})}{20,000}$$

$$= \frac{\overset{25}{\cancel{500,000}}}{\underset{1}{\cancel{20,000}}} = 25 \text{ mL/hr}$$

ANSWER: 25 mL per hr

EXAMPLE #2: The physician ordered 600 units per hr of heparin. You have available 1,000 mL of D5W with 25,000 units of heparin added. Calculate the flow rate in mL per hr. An infusion pump will be used.

Ratio and Proportion

25,000 units : 1,000 mL = 600 units : x mL
25,000x = 600,000 (1,000 × 600)

$$x = \frac{\overset{24}{\cancel{600,000}}}{\underset{1}{\cancel{25,000}}} = \frac{24}{1} = 24 \text{ mL/hr}$$

ANSWER: 24 mL per hr

The Formula Method

$$\frac{D}{H} \times Q = x$$

$$= \frac{600 \text{ units}}{25,000 \text{ units}} \times 1,000 \text{ mL} = x$$

$$\frac{600}{25,000} \times 1,000 \text{ mL} = \frac{\cancel{600,000}^{24}}{\cancel{25,000}_{1}}$$

$$= \frac{24}{1} = 24 \text{ mL/hr}$$

ANSWER: 24 mL per hr

Dimensional Analysis

$$\frac{600 \text{ units}}{hr} \times \frac{1,000 \text{ mL}}{25,000 \text{ units}}$$

$$\frac{600 \ \cancel{units}}{hr} \times \frac{1,000 \ (mL)}{25,000 \ \cancel{units}}$$

$$= \frac{600 \times 1,000 \ (mL)}{25,000} = \frac{\cancel{600,000}^{24}}{\cancel{25,000}_{1}}$$

$$= \frac{24}{1} = 24 \text{ mL/hr}$$

ANSWER: 24 mL per hr

Calculate Heparin Dosage (units per hr) When Heparin Is Ordered in Milliliters per Hour

RULE

To calculate units per hour when heparin is ordered in mL per hr: Calculate the desired hourly amount based on the available amount. Use one of the three standard methods of dosage calculation.

EXAMPLE: Give 1,000 mL of D5W with 30,000 units of heparin to infuse at 30 mL per hr. Calculate the hourly dosage of heparin.

Ratio and Proportion

30,000 units : 1,000 mL = x units : 30 mL
1,000x = 900,000 (30,000 × 30)

$$x = \frac{\overset{900}{\cancel{900,000}}}{\underset{1}{\cancel{1,000}}} = 900$$

x = 900 units/hr

ANSWER: 900 units per hr

The Formula Method

$$\frac{D}{H} \times Q = x$$

$$\frac{x \text{ units/hr}}{30,000} \times 1,000 \text{ mL} = 30 \text{ mL/hr}$$

1,000x = 900,000 (30 × 30,000)
x = 900 units/hr

ANSWER: 900 units per hr

Dimensional Analysis

$$\frac{30 \text{ mL}}{\text{hr}} \times \frac{300,00 \text{ units}}{1,000 \text{ mL}}$$

$$\frac{30 \text{ mL}}{\text{hr}} \times \frac{300,000 \text{ (units)}}{1,000 \text{ mL}}$$

$$= \frac{30 \times 300,000 \text{ (units)}}{1,000}$$

$$= \frac{900,000^{900}}{1,000_{1}} = \frac{900}{1}$$

$$= 900 \text{ units/hr}$$

Answer: 900 units per hr

Heparin Administration Based on Weight

Calculate Heparin Flow Rate (mL/hr) When Heparin Is Ordered Based on Weight (units/kg/hr)

RULE

To calculate the flow rate (mL/hr) when heparin is ordered in units/kg/hr: Convert to like units (lb to kg), calculate units/hr, and calculate mL/hr using one of the three standard methods to calculate dosages. The Formula Method is used here as an example.

| EXAMPLE: | A physician orders heparin 12,500 units in 250 mL D5W to run at 16 units/kg/hr for a patient weighing 124 lb. The nurse should set the infusion pump at ____ mL per hr. |

| CONVERT LB TO KG: | 124 lb ÷ 2.2 lb/kg = 56.4 kg
Round to the nearest tenth (56 kg) |

| CALCULATE UNITS/HR: | 16 units/kg/hr × 56 kg
= 896 units/hr |

| USE THE FORMULA METHOD: | $\dfrac{D}{H} \times Q = \text{mL/hr}$ |

| TO CALCULATE ML/HR: | $\dfrac{896 \text{ units/hr}}{12,500 \text{ units}} \times 250 \text{ mL} = x$ |

| SOLVE FOR X: | $x = 17.75$ or 18 mL/hr |

ANSWER: Set the infusion pump at 18 mL per hr

Calculate Heparin Dosage by Weight (units/kg/hr) When Heparin Is Ordered by Flow Rate (mL/hr)

RULE

To calculate units/kg/hr when the flow rate (mL/hr) is known: Convert to like units (lb to kg) and calculate the units/hr. Use one of the three standard methods of calculation. Ratio and Proportion will be used here.

EXAMPLE:	Heparin 12,500 units in 250 mL D5W is infusing at 15 mL per hr in a patient weighing 189 lb. How many units/kg/hr is the patient receiving?

CONVERT LB TO KG:	189 lb ÷ 2.2 lb/kg = 86 kg

CALCULATE UNITS/HR USING RATIO AND PROPORTION:	12,500 units : 250 mL = x units : 15 mL 250x = 187,000 (12,500 × 15) $x = \dfrac{187,500}{250} = 750$ units/hr

CALCULATE UNITS/KG/HR:	750 units/hr ÷ 86 kg = 8.7 units/kg/hr

ANSWER: 8.7 units/kg/hr

Weight-Based Heparin Protocol

Many hospitals now use standard protocols (guidelines) based on the patient's weight and blood results (PTT) to indicate a dosage range. The initial dose of heparin (bolus dose) is ordered in units per kg and is followed with a continuous intravenous infusion. The dosage of the infusion is adjusted over time based on the patient's continued response to heparin (PTT monitoring). The dosage is increased or decreased based on how close the blood levels are to the therapeutic PTT range. The hospital will provide a titration guideline for safe administration. Lovenox and Fragmin are examples of low-molecular-weight anticoagulants. See Table 13.1.

Table 13.1 **Weight-Based Heparin Protocol (DVT/PE)**

PTT less than 36	Give 80 units per kg as a bolus. Increase infusion rate by 4 units per kilogram per hour (4 U/kg/hr)
PTT 36 to 45	Give 40 units per kilogram as a bolus. Increase infusion rate by 2 units per kilogram per hour (2 U/kg/hr)
PTT 46 to 64	Increase infusion rate by 1 unit per kilogram per hour (1 U/kg/hr)
PTT 65 to 105	No change
PTT 106 to 120	Decrease infusion rate by 1 unit per kilogram per hour (1 U/kg/hr)
PTT 121 to 150	Decrease infusion rate by 2 units per kilogram per hour (2 U/kg/hr)
PTT greater than 150	Hold heparin for 1 hr and then decrease infusion rate by 3 units per kilogram per hour (3 U/kg/hr)

Reprinted with permission from The Chester County Hospital, West Chester, PA.

Calculate IV Heparin Flow Rate (mL/hr) When Heparin Is Ordered According to a Weight-Based Protocol

_R U L E_

To give heparin according to a protocol: Convert the patient's weight in pounds to kilograms, calculate the bolus dose (units), and calculate the infusion rate using one of the three standard methods of calculation. The Formula Method will be used here.

EXAMPLE #1: The physician prescribed 60 units per kg of a heparin bolus for a patient who weighs 110 lb. Heparin is available as 5,000 units per mL for a bolus dose. The infusion is ordered at 20 units/kg/hr. Heparin is available as 25,000 units per 500 mL NS. The nurse should give _____ mL as a bolus and set the infusion pump at _____ mL per hr.

CONVERT LB TO KG: 110 lb ÷ 2.2 lb/kg = 50 kg

CALCULATE BOLUS DOSE: 60 units/kg × 50 kg = 3,000 units
Heparin is available as 5,000 units/mL

USE THE FORMULA METHOD:
$$\frac{D}{H} \times Q = x$$

$$\frac{3,000 \text{ units}}{5,000 \text{ units}} \times 1 \text{ mL} = \frac{3}{5} \text{ mL} = 0.6 \text{ mL}$$

ANSWER: Give 0.6 mL for bolus dose.

START INFUSION: Start infusion at 20 units/kg/hr

CALCULATE ML/HR: Heparin is available as 25,000 units per 500 mL

USE THE FORMULA METHOD:
$$\frac{D}{H} \times Q = x$$

CALCULATE UNITS/HR: 20 units/kg/hr × 50 kg = 1,000 units/hr

CALCULATE mL/HR:	$$\frac{1{,}000 \text{ units/hr}}{25{,}000 \text{ units}} \times 500 \text{ mL} = 20 \text{ mL/hr}$$

ANSWER: Set pump at 20 mL per hr.

EXAMPLE #2:	A physician ordered heparin 12,500 units in 500 mL NS for a patient weighing 132 lb. Give a bolus dose of 80 units/kg (heparin is available as 10,000 units/mL) followed by an infusion of 20 units/kg/hr. The nurse should give ___ mL as a bolus dose and set the infusion pump at _____ mL per hr.

CONVERT LB TO KG:	132 lb ÷ 2.2 lb/kg = 60 kg

CALCULATE THE BOLUS DOSE:	80 units/kg × 60 kg = 4,800 units Heparin is available as 10,000 units

USE THE FORMULA METHOD TO CALCULATE BOLUS DOSE:	$$\frac{D}{H} \times Q = x$$ $$\frac{4{,}800 \text{ units}}{10{,}000 \text{ units}} \times 1 \text{ mL} = \frac{48}{100} = 0.48 \text{ mL}$$

ANSWER: Give 0.48 mL as a bolus dose.

START INFUSION:	20 units/kg/hr × 60 kg = 1,200 units/hr

CALCULATE mL/HR:

$$\frac{D}{H} \times Q = x$$

$$\frac{1{,}200 \text{ units/hr}}{12{,}500 \text{ units}} \times 500 \text{ mL} = x$$

$$\frac{1{,}200 \times 500}{12{,}500} = \frac{\cancel{600{,}000}^{\,48}}{\cancel{12{,}500}_{\,1}}$$

$$= \frac{48}{1} = 48 \text{ mL/hr}$$

ANSWER: Set the infusion pump at 48 mL per hr.

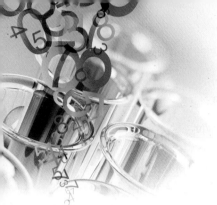

Complete the following problems:

1. Give 500 mL of D5 NS with 10,000 units of
   heparin to infuse at 20 mL per hr. Calculate the
   hourly dosage of heparin. Is the dosage within
   the normal, safe range for 24 hr?
   Answer = _____ units per hr. Safe
   or unsafe? _____

2. Give 1,000 mL of D5W with 10,000 units of
   heparin IV over 24 hr. Is the dosage within the
   normal, safe range for 24 hr? _____

3. Give 800 units of heparin IV every hour. You
   have 1,000 mL of D5 NS with 40,000 units of
   heparin added. Calculate the flow rate.
   Answer = _____ mL per hr

4. The physician prescribes a heparin bolus of
   80 units per kg followed by an infusion of
   heparin 12,500 units in 250 mL D5W to run
   at 18 units/kg/hr in a patient weighing 56 kg.
   You should administer _____ units IV push
   for the bolus and start the infusion at _____
   mL per hr.

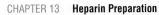

5. The results of a PTT blood test came back for the patient in Question #4. The protocol directs you to increase the infusion by 2 units/kg/hr. After recalculating the rate you set the infusion pump at _____ mL per hr.

> ### Critical Thinking Check
>
> Since the infusion was increased, can you assume that the patient's PTT result was equal to, greater than, or less than the previous reading and the control? _____ **Equal to, Less Than, or Greater Than?**

6. Heparin 12,500 units in 250 mL D5W is infusing at 21 mL per hr in a patient who weighs 92 kg. How many units per kilogram per hour is the patient receiving at this flow rate? _____

7. A patient is to receive 10,000 units of heparin subcutaneously at 8:00 AM and 8:00 PM for 5 days. Heparin sodium for injection is available in a TUBEX Cartridge-Needle unit in 15,000 units per mL. The nurse should give _____ mL every 12 hr for a daily total dosage of _____ units per 24 hr. This is/is not within the normal dosage range. _____

8. Heparin sodium, 8,000 units, is to be given subcutaneously every 8 hr. The medication is available in a vial labeled 10,000 units per milliliter. The nurse should give _____ mL every 8 hr for a total dosage of _____ units per 24 hr. This is/is not within the normal dosage range. _____

> ## Critical Thinking Check
>
> If an alternate dosage was prescribed for this patient, which daily dosage would you recognize as unsafe to give: _____ **10,000 units per 8 hr; 12,000 units per 8 hr; or 15,000 units per 8 hr?**

9. The physician prescribed heparin sodium, 5,000 units, subcutaneously twice a day. Heparin is available in a vial labeled 7,500 units per milliliter. The nurse should give _____ mL twice a day for a total dosage of _____ units per 24 hr. This is/is not within the normal dosage range. _____

10. The physician prescribed 5,000 units of heparin for injection intravenously through a heparin lock. Heparin is available in a 10-mL vial in a concentration of 20,000 units per milliliter. The nurse should administer _____ mL.

11. The physician ordered 500 mL of D5W with 30,000 units of heparin to infuse at 10 mL per hr. Calculate the hourly dosage of heparin: _____ units per hr in 10 mL.

12. The physician prescribed 1,000 mL of 0.45% NS with 15,000 units of heparin IV, every 8 hours. Calculate the units per 24 hr: _____; safe or unsafe range? _____.

13. You are to give 500 units of heparin IV hourly. You have 1,000 mL D5W with 10,000 units of heparin added. Calculate the flow rate: _____ mL per hr.

14. A patient is to receive 500 mL of D5W with 15,000 units of heparin over 24 hr. Using an infusion pump, the nurse should set the flow rate at _____ mL per hr to deliver _____ units per hr of heparin.

15. The activated PTT is elevated and the protocol directs you to hold the heparin (12,500 units in 250 mL D5W) infusion for 1 hr and restart it at 10 units/kg/hr. If the patient weighs 140 lb, how many mL per hr should the patient receive? _____

16. Heparin 12,500 units in 250 mL D5W is infusing at 15 mL per hr in a patient weighing 126 lb. You would document that the patient is receiving _____ units per kilogram per hour.

thePoint, Additional practice problems to enhance learning and facilitate chapter comprehension can be found on **http://thePoint.lww.com/Boyer8e.**

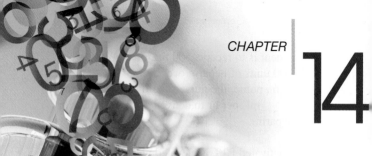

14

Pediatric Dosage Calculations and Intravenous Therapy

LEARNING OBJECTIVES

After completing this chapter, you should be able to:

- Convert weight in pounds to kilograms, kilograms to pounds, and grams to kilograms.
- Calculate the lower and upper safe dosage ranges and total daily safe dosage.
- Estimate body surface area using a nomogram and a formula.
- Calculate oral and parenteral dosages based on body weight (mg/kg).
- Calculate oral and parenteral dosages using body surface area (BSA).
- Calculate intravenous flow rate.

• Calculate intermittent intravenous medication administration (intravenous piggyback [IVPB]).
• Explain how to deliver IV push medications.

*E*xtreme care must be taken when preparing and administering medications to infants (birth to 12 months), children (1 to 12 years), and adolescents (13 to 18 years). Because there are such variations among children (size, weight, maturity of system, and medication rates of absorption), only two methods are currently used to calculate pediatric dosages. Dosages are calculated by either using body weight (mg/kg) or body surface area (BSA), which is measured in square meters (m^2). Therefore, you need to become comfortable converting pounds to kilograms (1 kg = 2.2 lb), grams to kilograms (1,000 g = 1 kg), and micrograms to milligrams (1,000 mcg = 1 mg) and using a nomogram. The West nomogram is shown in Figure 14.1.

A nurse *must always determine that the ordered dosage is safe* before administering the medication! *Always compare the prescribed dosage to the recommended safe dosage range using a reference drug resource when calculating dosages.* You should also use a calculator to double-check your calculations.

Oral pediatric medications are prescribed in liquid form whenever possible. It is best to use a syringe or dropper to give medications to infants and toddlers; a cup can be used for school-age children. *Parenteral* medications are most commonly given subcutaneously (upper arm, abdomen, and thigh) for immunizations and insulin and intramuscularly (vastus lateralis for infants and the gluteus after toddlers start walking) for vaccines. Dosage amounts are limited to 1 mL per site for those younger than 5 years of age (usually

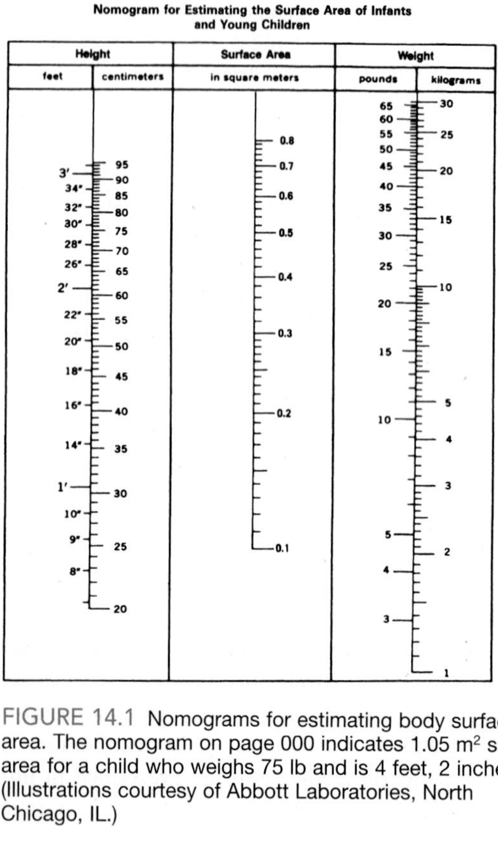

FIGURE 14.1 Nomograms for estimating body surface area. The nomogram on page 000 indicates 1.05 m² surface area for a child who weighs 75 lb and is 4 feet, 2 inches tall. (Illustrations courtesy of Abbott Laboratories, North Chicago, IL.)

0.5 mL for infants), and the quantity is measured using a tuberculin syringe. Children ages 6 to 12 years can be given up to 2 mL of solution per site; the volume limit for adolescents is 3 mL per site. Refer to Appendix E for information on subcutaneous injections and Appendix H for pediatric intramuscular

**Nomogram for Estimating the Surface Area
of Older Children and Adults**

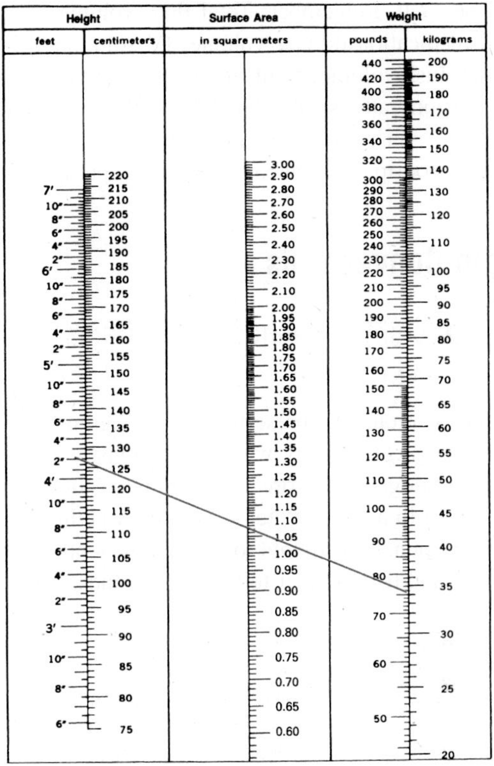

Height		Surface Area	Weight	
feet	centimeters	in square meters	pounds	kilograms

FIGURE 14.1 (*continued*)

injections. Appendix I covers nursing concerns for
pediatric drug administration.

It is essential that pediatric *intravenous* therapy
be as exact as possible because infants and children
have a narrow range of fluid balance. Therefore, a

microdrip, volume-controlled set (Buretrol) or a pump should be used. Remember: Total fluid volume consists of medication diluent volume, IV solution volume, and flush volume (5 mL to 20 mL). An intravenous infusion rate is calculated in both drops per minute (i.e., via a Buretrol) and milliliters per hour using a microdrip or an electronic infusion pump.

Weight Conversions

Convert Weight in Pounds to Kilograms and Kilograms to Pounds

When medications are prescribed in milligrams per kilogram (mg/kg) of body weight, you must convert pounds to kilograms before calculating the dosage. There are 2.2 lb in 1 kg. Note: If a child's weight is in pounds and ounces, estimate to the nearest tenth of a pound and add that number to the total pounds.

RULE

To convert pounds to kilograms: *Divide* the patient's body weight in pounds by 2.2. To convert kilograms to pounds: *Multiply* the patient's body weight in kilograms by 2.2. *Note:* For premature infants, you will probably need to work with grams (1,000 g = 1 kg). Use one of these three methods for calculation of dosages: simple division or multiplication, ratio and proportion, or dimensional analysis.

EXAMPLE #1:   Convert a child's weight of 44 lb into kilograms.

Basic Division

Move the decimal point in the divisor and the dividend the same number of places. Put the decimal point directly above the line for the quotient.

$$2.2.\overline{)44.0.}$$

$$\begin{array}{r} 20. \text{ (quotient)} \\ 22\overline{)440.} \end{array}$$

ANSWER: 20 kg

Ratio and Proportion

2.2 lb : 1 kg = 44 lb : x kg
2.2x = 44

$$x = \frac{44}{2.2} = \frac{\cancel{440}^{20}}{\cancel{22}_1} = \frac{20}{1} = 20$$

ANSWER: 20 kg

Note: Move the decimal point in the denominator and the numerator the same number of spaces prior to doing the cancellation.

Dimensional Analysis

$$\frac{44 \text{ lb}}{} \times \frac{1 \text{ kg}}{2.2 \text{ lb}}$$

$$= \frac{44 \cancel{\text{ lb}}}{} \times \frac{1 \text{ kg}}{2.2 \cancel{\text{ lb}}} = \frac{44 \times 1 \text{ (kg)}}{2.2}$$

$$= \frac{\cancel{440}^{20}}{\cancel{22}_1} = \frac{20}{1} = 20$$

ANSWER: 20 kg

Note: Move the decimal point in the denominator and the numerator the same number of spaces prior to doing the cancellation.

EXAMPLE #2: Convert a child's weight of 25 kg to pounds.

Basic Multiplication

$$2.2 \text{ lb} \times 25 \text{ kg/lb} = 55 \text{ lb}$$

ANSWER: 55 lb

Ratio and Proportion

$$2.2 \text{ lb} : 1 \text{ kg} = x \text{ lb} : 25 \text{ kg}$$
$$x = 25 \times 2.2$$
$$x = 55 \text{ pounds}$$

ANSWER: 55 lb

Dimensional Analysis

$$\frac{25 \text{ kg}}{} \times \frac{2.2 \text{ lb}}{1 \text{ kg}}$$

$$= \frac{25 \ \cancel{\text{kg}}}{} \times \frac{2.2 \ (\text{lb})}{1 \ \cancel{\text{kg}}} = \frac{25 \times 2.2}{1} = 55$$

ANSWER: 55 lb

Convert Weight in Grams to Kilograms

RULE

To convert grams to kilograms for infants: Divide the infant's body weight (in grams) by 1,000 and round to the nearest tenth.

| EXAMPLE: | Convert an infant's weight of 2,270 g to kilograms. |

Ratio and Proportion

$1 \text{ kg} : 1,000 \text{ g} = x \text{ kg} : 2,270 \text{ g}$
$1,000x = 2,270$

$$x = \frac{2,270}{1,000} = 2.27 \text{ kg}$$

ANSWER: 2.3 kg

Dimensional Analysis

$$\frac{2,270 \text{ g}}{} \times \frac{1 \text{ kg}}{1,000 \text{ g}}$$

$$\frac{2,270 \text{ g}}{} \times \frac{1 \text{ kg}}{1,000 \text{ g}} = \frac{2,270 \times 1 \text{ (kg)}}{1,000}$$

$$= \frac{2,270}{1,000} = 2.27$$

ANSWER: 2.3 kg

Estimate Safe Total Daily Dosage

Pediatric medications have an upper and a lower safe dosage range used to indicate a safe, total daily dose. You can find this information on the drug package insert, a drug reference, or an institutional protocol. You need this information before you calculate any dose to give to a child.

RULE

To calculate safe, total, daily dosage: Multiply the patient's weight in kilograms by the recommended dosage in milligrams.

EXAMPLE #1: A child weighs 15 kg. The safe daily drug dosage is 4 mg/kg/day.

Estimate Total Daily Dosage

4 mg × 15 kg = 60 mg/day

> ***ANSWER:*** Total daily dosage = 60 mg per day

EXAMPLE #2: A child weighs 20 kg. The physician orders 10 mg of a drug every 6 hr. The safe daily dosage is 2.5 mg/kg/day.

Estimate Total Daily Dosage

10 mg × 4 doses = 40 mg/day
(24 hr ÷ 6 = 4 doses/day)

Determine If the Prescribed Dose Is Safe

Safe dosage is: 2.5 mg/kg/day
Estimate: 2.5 mg × 20 kg = 50 mg, divided into
> 4 doses = 12.5 mg/dose
Determine: Dose of 10 mg, q6h, is safe.

RULE

To calculate the safe lower and upper dosage range: Multiply the child's weight in kilograms by the lower and upper dosage ranges in milligrams: milligrams per kilogram per day (mg/kg/day) or milligrams per kilogram per dose (mg/kg/dose).

EXAMPLE:	A physician orders 75 mg of an antibiotic, q8h, for a child who weighs 30 kg. The safe dosage range is 6 to 8 mg/kg/day. Calculate the lower and upper dosage ranges.
ESTIMATE TOTAL DAILY DOSAGE:	75 mg × 3 doses (24 hr ÷ 8 hr) = 225 mg
CALCULATE LOWER DOSE RANGE:	6 mg/kg/day × 30 kg = 180 mg
CALCULATE UPPER DOSE RANGE:	8 mg/kg/day × 30 kg = 240 mg
DETERMINE IF DOSE IS SAFE:	Yes. The total daily dosage of 225 mg is safe.

Calculate Oral and Parenteral Dosages Based on Body Weight (mg per kg)

RULE

To calculate dosage based on body weight: *Convert* pounds to kilograms (divide by 2.2), *calculate* safe dosage range, *compare* the prescribed dosage with the safe dosage range, and *calculate* the dose needed using one of three calculation methods. Remember the sequence of activities: *convert, calculate, compare, and calculate!*

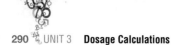
EXAMPLE #1: The physician prescribed an antibiotic, 20 mg/kg/day, PO. The patient weighs 44 lb. The antibiotic is available as 250 mg per 10 mL. The safe dosage range for the antibiotic is 20 to 40 mg/kg/day. The nurse should give x mL, twice daily.

CONVERT: 44 lb to kilograms
44 lb ÷ 2.2 lb/kg = 20 kg

CALCULATE SAFE DOSAGE: The safe dosage range is 20 to 40 mg/kg/day.
20 kg × 20 mg (low range) = 400 mg
20 kg × 40 mg (high range) = 800 mg
The safe dosage range for this child is 400 to 800 mg per day.

COMPARE PRESCRIBED DOSE WITH SAFE DOSE: The prescribed dose is 20 mg/kg/day or 400 mg daily.
This dose is within the lower range of safe dosage.
Therefore, it is a safe dose to give.

CALCULATE THE DOSE: Calculate mL to give by using one of the three calculation methods.

Ratio and Proportion

250 mg : 10 mL = 400 mg : x mL
250x = 4,000

$$x = \frac{4,000^{16}}{250_1} = \frac{16}{1} = 16 \text{ mL}$$

ANSWER: 16 mL

The Formula Method

$$\text{Use } \frac{D}{H} \times Q = x$$

$$\frac{400 \text{ mg}}{250 \text{ mg}} \times 10 \text{ mL} = x$$

$$\frac{400}{250} \times 10 \text{ mL} = \frac{4{,}000^{16}}{250_1} = \frac{16}{1} = 16 \text{ mL}$$

ANSWER: 16 mL

Dimensional Analysis

$$\frac{400 \text{ mg}}{} = \frac{10 \text{ mL}}{250 \text{ mg}}$$

$$\frac{400 \text{ mg}}{} = \frac{10 \text{ (mL)}}{250 \text{ mg}} = \frac{400 \times 10 \text{ (mL)}}{250}$$

$$= \frac{4{,}000^{16}}{250_1} = \frac{16}{1} = 16 \text{ mL}$$

ANSWER: 16 mL

EXAMPLE #2: The physician prescribed 125 mg of an antibiotic, PO, q8h for a 33-lb child. The antibiotic is available as 250 mg per 5 mL. The safe dosage range is 20 to 40 mg/kg/ day. The nurse should give x mL, three times daily.

CONVERT: 33 lb to kilograms
33 lb ÷ 2.2 lb/kg = 15 kg.

CALCULATE
SAFE DOSAGE:

The safe dosage range is 20 to 40 mg/
kg/day.
15 kg × 20 mg (low range) = 300 mg
15 kg × 40 mg (high range) = 600 mg
The safe dosage range for this child is
300 to 600 mg per day.

COMPARE
PRESCRIBED
DOSE WITH
SAFE DOSE:

The prescribed dose is 125 mg, q8h,
or 375 mg daily.
This dose is within the safe dosage range.
Therefore, it is a safe dose to give.

CALCULATE
THE DOSE:

Calculate mL to give by using one of the
three calculation methods.

Ratio and Proportion

125 mg : x mL = 250 mg : 5 mL
250x = 625 (5 × 125)

$$x = \frac{625}{250} = 2.5 \text{ mL}$$

ANSWER: 2.5 mL per 8 hr

The Formula Method

$$\text{Use } \frac{D}{H} \times Q = x$$

$$\frac{125 \text{ mg}}{250 \text{ mg}} \times 5 = x$$

$$\frac{\overset{1}{\cancel{125}}}{\underset{2}{\cancel{250}}} \times 5 = \frac{5}{2} = 2.5 \text{ mL}$$

ANSWER: 2.5 mL per 8 hr

Dimensional Analysis

$$\frac{125 \text{ mg}}{} \times \frac{5 \text{ mL}}{250 \text{ mg}}$$

$$\frac{125 \text{ mg}}{} \times \frac{5 \text{ (mL)}}{250 \text{ mg}} = \frac{125 \times 5 \text{ (mL)}}{250}$$

$$= \frac{625}{250} = 2.5 \text{ mL}$$

ANSWER: 2.5 mL per 8 hr

Estimate Body Surface Area

Estimating body surface area (BSA), in square meters (m^2), is the most accurate way of calculating drug dosages. There are two ways to estimate BSA. You can use a chart—the West nomogram (Figure 14.1)—or a formula that uses the metric system but requires a calculator that can perform the square root function.

EXAMPLE #1: A child weighs 24 lb and is 36 inches tall. To estimate BSA, draw a line from the weight of 24 lb and the height of 36 inches. The line will intersect at 0.5 m^2.

ANSWER: BSA = 0.5 m^2

EXAMPLE #2: A child weighs 50 lb and has a height of 40 inches. What is the BSA?

USE THIS FORMULA:

$$\sqrt{\frac{\text{Weight (kg)} \times \text{height (cm)}}{3,600}} = x$$

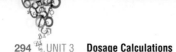

TAKE THE SQUARE ROOT:	$\sqrt{x} = \text{BSA}$

CONVERT 50 LB TO KILOGRAMS:	1 kg = 2.2 lb 50 lb ÷ 2.2 lb/kg = 22.7 kg

CONVERT 40 INCHES TO CENTIMETERS:	1 inch = 2.5 cm 40 inches × 2.5 cm/inch = 100 cm

APPLY FORMULA:

$$\sqrt{\frac{22.7\ (\text{kg}) \times 100\ (\text{cm})}{3,600}} = \frac{2,270}{3,600} = 0.63$$

TAKE SQUARE ROOT:

$$\sqrt{0.63}$$

ANSWER: BSA = 0.79

Dosage Calculations Based on Body Surface Area

There are two rules that can be used. Rule #2 is the most accurate approach.

RULE #1

To calculate a safe child's dosage when you only have the average adult dose: Estimate the child's BSA, divide the child's BSA in square meters (m^2) by 1.73 m^2 (surface area of an average adult), and multiply by the adult dose.

EXAMPLE #1:   The physician prescribed Benadryl for an 8-year-old child who weighs 75 lb and is 50 inches tall (4 feet, 2 inches). The normal adult dose is 25 mg, q.i.d. The nurse should give x mg, q.i.d. A straight line drawn from height to weight, using the West nomogram, intersects at 1.05 m².

USE BODY SURFACE AREA RULE:

$$\frac{\text{Child's BSA}}{1.73 \text{ m}^2} \times \text{adult dose}$$

$$\frac{1.05 \text{ m}^2}{1.73 \text{ m}^2} = 0.06 \times 25 \text{ mg} = 15.17 \text{ mg}$$

ANSWER: 15 mg, q.i.d.

RULE #2

To calculate a safe child's dosage: Determine the patient's BSA (m²), calculate the safe dosage in mg/m²/dose using a reference, decide if the prescribed dose is within the safe dosage range, and calculate the dose needed using one of the three calculation methods.

EXAMPLE #2:   The physician prescribed 2.5 mg of an antibiotic, PO, twice daily, for 5 days for a child who is 34 inches tall and weighs 25 lb. The medication is available as a scored 5-mg tablet. The medication label lists a safe dosage range of 10 mg/m²/day. The nurse should give x tablets per dose.

DETERMINE BSA: Draw a straight line from the height of 34 inches to the weight of 25 lb. The line intersects at 0.5 m².

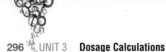
CALCULATE SAFE DOSAGE:	The safe dosage range is 10 mg/m²/day $10 \text{ mg} \times 0.5 \text{ m}^2 = 5 \text{ mg/day}$
COMPARE PRESCRIBED DOSE WITH SAFE DOSE:	The prescribed dose is 2.5 mg, q12h, which falls within the safe dosage range of 5 mg per day. Therefore, it is a safe dose to give.
CALCULATE THE DOSE:	Solve for x using one of the three calculation methods.

Ratio and Proportion

5 mg : 1 tablet = 2.5 mg : x
$5x = 2.5$

$$x = \frac{\cancel{2.5}^{1}}{\cancel{5}_{2}} = \frac{1}{2} \text{ tablet}$$

ANSWER: ½ tablet, q12h

The Formula Method

$$\frac{D}{H} \times Q = x$$

$$\frac{2.5 \text{ mg}}{5 \text{ mg}} \times 1 \text{ tablet} = x$$

$$\frac{\cancel{2.5}^{1}}{\cancel{5}_{2}} = \frac{1}{2} \text{ tablet}$$

ANSWER: ½ tablet, q12h

Dimensional Analysis

$$\frac{2.5 \text{ mg}}{} \times \frac{1 \text{ tablet}}{5 \text{ mg}}$$

$$= \frac{2.5 \text{ mg}}{} \times \frac{1 \text{ tablet}}{5 \text{ mg}} = \frac{2.5 \times 1 \text{ (tablet)}}{5}$$

$$= \frac{2.5^{1}}{5_{2}} = \frac{1}{2} \text{ tablet}$$

ANSWER: ½ tablet, q12h

PRACTICE PROBLEMS

1. A physician prescribed Biaxin 275 mg, PO, q8h, for a 44-lb child with pneumonia. The safe dosage is 15 mg/kg/day. If the nurse gave 275 mg per dose, would this be a safe daily dose? Yes _____ or No _____

2. A physician prescribed codeine 30 mg, q4h, as needed, for a child in pain. The child weighs 44 lb. The safe dosage is 5 to 10 mg/kg/dose. If the nurse gave 30 mg per dose, six times a day, would this be a safe dose? Yes _____ or No _____

3. An emergency department physician ordered 4 mg of a drug for a 44-lb child with a seizure. The safe dosage range is 0.04 to 0.2 mg/kg/dose. The nurse gave _____ mg. Is this a safe dose? Yes _____ or No _____

4. The physician ordered Augmentin Suspension 550 mg, PO, q8h, for a child with otitis media. Augmentin is labeled 250 mg per 5 mL. The nurse should administer _____ mL, q8h.

5. The physician prescribed 60 mg of a drug, PO, q6h, for an 88-lb child. The child weighs _____ kg. The safe dosage range is 5 to 7 mg/kg/day. Therefore, the safe dosage range for this child is _____ mg per dose. If the nurse gave 60 mg per dose, would this be a safe dose? Yes _____ or No _____

6. The physician prescribed nafcillin 1 g, q6h, for a 132-lb teenager. The teenager weighs _____ kg. The safe dosage range is 50 to 100 mg/kg/day. Therefore, the safe dosage range for this teenager is _____ g/day. If the nurse gave 1 g per dose, would this be safe? Yes _____ or No _____

7. A physician ordered penicillin V potassium 375 mg, PO, q6h, for a 66-lb child. The child weighs _____ kg. The safe dosage range is 25 to 50 mg/kg/24 hr. The dosage range for this child is _____ mg per day. Is this a safe dose? Yes _____ or No _____

8. A physician prescribed Dilantin 50 mg, PO, q12h, for a 33-lb child with a seizure disorder. The child weighs _____ kg. The safe dosage range is 5 to 10 mg/kg/day. The dosage range for this child is _____ mg per day. Is this a safe dose? Yes _____ or No _____

9. A physician ordered Orapred liquid 20 mg, PO,
q12h, for a 44-lb child. The child weighs
_____ kg. The safe dosage range is 0.5 to
2 mg/kg/day. The safe dosage range for this child
is _____ mg per day. Orapred liquid is
labeled as 5 mg per mL. The nurse would give
_____ mL per dose. Is this a safe dose? Yes _____
or No _____

10. The physician ordered ranitidine HCl 15 mg, PO,
q12h, for a 5-kg infant with gastroesophageal
reflux disease (GERD). The safe dosage range is
5 to 10 mg/kg/day. The safe dosage range for
this child is _____ mg per day. If the nurse gave
30 mg per day, would this be a safe dose?
Yes _____ or No _____

11. A physician prescribed Accutane 50 mg, PO,
twice a day, for acne for a 110-lb teenager. The
safe dosage range is 0.5 to 2 mg/kg/day. The safe
dosage range for this teenager is _____ mg per
day. If the nurse gave 50 mg per dose, would this
be a safe dose? Yes _____ or No _____

12. The physician prescribed Tylenol drops 100 mg,
PO, q4h, p.r.n., for temperature greater than
101.4°F for an infant who weighs 8 kg. Tylenol
drops are available as 80 mg per 0.8 mL. The
safe dosage range is 10 to 15 mg/kg/dose. The
dosage range for this infant is _____ mg per
dose. The nurse would give _____ mL of
Tylenol. Is this a safe dose? Yes _____ or
No _____

13. The physician prescribed Ceclor 200 mg, PO, every 8 hr, for a 33-lb toddler. The safe dosage range is 20 to 40 mg/kg/day. The dosage range for this toddler is _____ mg per day. Is this a safe dose? Yes _____ or No _____

Critical Thinking Check

If the physician increased the dosage of Ceclor to 300 mg per 8 hr, would the dosage be within a safe range to give? _____ **Yes or No?**

---

14. A 4-year-old is prescribed one dose of Rocephin 300 mg, IM. The label on the vial is Rocephin 500 mg per 2.5 mL. You should administer _____ mL.

15. Using BSA, calculate a physician order of Tylenol drops for a 6-year-old who weighs 50 lb and is 36 inches tall. The normal adult dose is 650 mg. The child's BSA = _____ m². The nurse should administer _____ mg each dose. Tylenol drops are available as labeled 80 mg per 0.8 mL. The nurse should administer _____ mL.

Calculate Intravenous Flow Rate

An infusion pump or volume-controlled unit is always used for pediatric intravenous therapy to reduce the possibility of fluid overload. The volume-controlled unit (e.g., Buretrol) is used when the total volume is less than 150 mL. The primary caution in administering IV medications to pediatric patients is the amount of *fluid volume* that is used.

IV tubing with a drop factor of 60 gtt per mL is recommended (required for infants and small children) because the amount of IV volume is less than that prescribed for adults. The guidelines for regulating flow rate and mL/hr using a pump or control unit are the same for a child as for an adult (see Chapter 10). However, with children, the rates must be closely monitored to prevent fluid overload. It is essential that pediatric intravenous therapy be as exact as possible because infants and children have a narrow range of fluid balance.

| EXAMPLE: | Give 200 mL of NS over 4 hr to a 5-year-old child. An infusion pump is used. |

| USE THIS FORMULA: |

$$\frac{\text{Total volume}}{\text{Total time (minutes)}} = \frac{x \ (\text{mL/hr})}{60 \ \text{min}}$$

$$\frac{200 \ \text{mL}}{240 \ \text{min}} = \frac{x \ (\text{mL/hr})}{60 \ \text{min}}$$

$$240x = 12{,}000$$

$$x = \frac{12{,}000}{240}$$

$$x = 50 \ \text{mL/hr}$$

ANSWER: Set pump to deliver 50 mL per hr

Calculate Intermittent Intravenous Medication Administration (Intravenous Piggyback: IVPB)

Dosages for IV medications are based on weight and calculated in mg per kg. Most drugs are available in a powder that comes premixed and has to be reconstituted (diluted) using a prescribed type and amount of diluent. Always follow the manufacturer's dilution requirements! Some institutions provide standard guidelines to assist the nurse in preparing IV pediatric dosages. Additional information about IVPB delivery can be found in Chapter 10.

Buretrols, Solusets, or other volume-controlled infusion sets/pumps are always used to regulate the infusion. These control devices reduce the possibility of fluid overload. *Always remember!* When administering IV medications, the total fluid volume consists of medication diluent volume, IV solution volume, and flush volume (5 to 10 mL). See Figure 14.2.

RULE

To calculate an IVPB medication:
- Convert the child's weight from pounds to kilograms.
- Calculate the safe dosage range. Use a reference.
- Compare the prescribed dose of medication with the safe dosage.
- Verify the type and amount of diluent for reconstitution.
- Calculate the amount of medication to be given.
- Add IV solution and medication to Buretrol.
- Calculate the flow rate and set the pump to mL per hr.
- Flush tubing with 5 mL to 20 mL of flush solution and chart fluid intake. Follow institutional guidelines for IV flush.

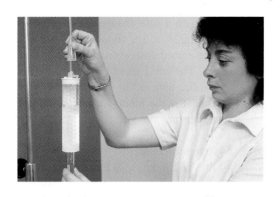

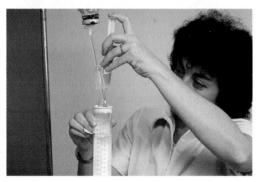

FIGURE 14.2 Volume-controlled set. (From Taylor, C., Lillis, C., and LeMone, P. [2008]. *Fundamentals of nursing: The art and science of nursing care* [6th ed.]. Philadelphia: Lippincott Williams & Wilkins.)

EXAMPLE #1: The physician prescribed 125 mg of an antibiotic to be given, IV, via a Buretrol, q6h, in 50 mL of NS to infuse over 30 min. Follow with a 10-mL NS flush. The antibiotic is available as 250 mg per

4 mL with a safe dosage range of 25 to 50 mg/kg/24 hr. The child weighs 44 lb. Is the prescribed dose within the safe dosage range? The nurse should give x mL of the antibiotic, q6h, in 50 mL of D5W over 30 min. Set the pump for a flow rate of x mL per hr.

CONVERT:	44 lb to kilograms 44 lb ÷ 2.2 lb/kg = 20 kg

CALCULATE SAFE DOSAGE:	The safe dosage range is 25 to 50 mg/kg/day. 25 mg (lower range) × 20 kg = 500 mg 50 mg (upper range) × 20 kg = 1,000 mg

COMPARE PRESCRIBED DOSE WITH THE SAFE DOSE:	The safe dosage range for this child is 500 to 1,000 mg/day The prescribed dose is 125 mg, q6h, which equals 500 mg per day. Therefore, the prescribed dosage is within the safe dosage range.

CALCULATE THE DOSE:	Solve for x using one of the three calculation methods.

Ratio and Proportion

250 mg : 4 mL = 125 mg : x mL
$250x = 500 \ (125 \times 2)$

$$x = \frac{\cancel{500}^{2}}{\cancel{250}_{1}} = \frac{2}{1} = 2 \text{ mL}$$

ANSWER: $x = 2$ mL

The Formula Method

$$\frac{D}{H} \times Q = x$$

$$\frac{125 \text{ mg}}{250 \text{ mg}} \times 4 \text{ mL} = x$$

$$x = \frac{125 \times 4}{250} = \frac{\overset{2}{\cancel{500}}}{\underset{1}{\cancel{250}}} = \frac{2}{1} = 2 \text{ mL}$$

ANSWER: $x = 2$ mL

Dimensional Analysis

$$\frac{125 \cancel{\text{ mg}}}{} \times \frac{4 \text{ mL}}{250 \cancel{\text{ mg}}}$$

$$\frac{125}{} \times \frac{4 \text{ (mL)}}{250} = \frac{4 \text{ (mL)} \times 125}{250}$$

$$= \frac{\overset{2}{\cancel{500}}}{\underset{1}{\cancel{250}}} = \frac{2}{1} = 2 \text{ mL}$$

ANSWER: $x = 2$ mL

ADD IV SOLUTION: To give 125 mg, you would prepare 2 mL of the antibiotic. Allow 48 mL of NS to run into the Buretrol and then add 2 mL of the antibiotic.

CALCULATE THE FLOW RATE: Use the Standard Formula to determine mL/hr.

$$\frac{\text{Total volume} \times \text{Drop factor}}{\text{Total time in minutes}} = \text{mL/hr}$$

$$\frac{50 \times 60}{30} = \frac{3,000}{30} = 100 \text{ mL/hr}$$

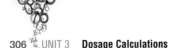
SET THE PUMP:	To deliver 125 mg in 50 mL NS, set the pump to 100 mL/hr.
FLUSH TUBING:	Flush the tubing with 10 mL of NS.
CHART FLUID INTAKE:	Chart the intake of 60 mL (48 + 2 + 10).

EXAMPLE #2:	A 4-year old child who weighs 55 lb is prescribed 250 mg of an antibiotic to be given IVPB, via a Buretrol, in 50 mL of NSS, q6h. The safe dosage range is 30 to 60 mg/kg/24 hr. Infuse over 30 min. The antibiotic is available as a powder labeled 500 mg. To dilute, add 2 mL of sterile water for a solution of 200 mg per mL. Use 20 mL as a flush solution. The Buretrol is connected to a pump.
CONVERT:	55 lb to kilograms 55 lb ÷ 2.2 lb/kg = 25 kg
CALCULATE SAFE DOSAGE:	The safe dosage range is 30 to 60 mg/kg/24 hr 25 kg × 30 mg (low range) = 750 mg 25 kg × 60 mg (high range) = 1,500 mg The safe dosage range for this child is 750 to 1,500 mg/day
COMPARE PRESCRIBED DOSE WITH SAFE DOSE:	The prescribed dose is 250 mg, q6h, or 1,000 mg daily. This dose is within the safe dosage range. Therefore, it is a safe dose to give.
VERIFY AMOUNT OF DILUENT:	Add 2 mL of sterile water to the vial for a solution of 200 mg/mL.

CALCULATE THE DOSE:	Solve for x using one of the three calculation methods.

Ratio and Proportion

250 mg : x = 200 mg : 1 mL
200x = 250

$$x = \frac{\cancel{250}^{5}}{\cancel{200}_{4}} = \frac{5}{4} = 1.25 \text{ mL}$$

ANSWER: 1.25 mL

The Formula Method

$$\frac{D}{H} \times Q = x$$

$$\frac{250 \text{ mg}}{200 \text{ mg}} \times 1 \text{ mL} = x$$

$$\frac{\cancel{250}^{5}}{\cancel{200}_{4}} = \frac{5}{4} = 1.25 \text{ mL}$$

ANSWER: 1.25 mL

Dimensional Analysis

$$\frac{250 \text{ mg}}{} \times \frac{1 \text{ mL}}{200 \text{ mg}}$$

$$\frac{250 \cancel{\text{ mg}}}{} \times \frac{1 \text{ (mL)}}{200 \cancel{\text{ mg}}} = \frac{250 \times 1 \text{ (mL)}}{200}$$

$$= \frac{\cancel{250}^{5}}{\cancel{200}_{4}} = \frac{5}{4} = 1.25 \text{ mL}$$

ANSWER: 1.25 mL

ADD IV SOLUTION:	Add 48.75 mL of NSS plus 1.25 mL of medication to the Buretrol.
CALCULATE THE FLOW RATE:	Use the standard formula. When the infusion time is less than 60 min, add 60 min as a conversion factor.

$$\frac{\text{Total volume}}{\text{Total time in minutes}} = \frac{\text{mL/hr}}{60 \text{ min}}$$

$$\frac{50 \text{ mL}}{30 \text{ min}} = \frac{x \text{ mL}}{60 \text{ min}}$$

$$30x = 3,000$$

$$x = 100 \text{ mL}$$

SET THE PUMP:	Set the infusion pump to 100 mL/hr. The pump will deliver 50 mL in 30 min.
FLUSH TUBING:	Flush the tubing with 20 mL of NSS.
CHART FLUID INTAKE:	Chart an intake of 70 mL (48.75 + 1.25 + 20)

Calculate IV Push Medications

To calculate the amount of medication to prepare for an IV push delivery, follow the first five steps in the foregoing rule. Because you would be pushing the medication into the vein, your next step would be to determine, from the order or a standard reference, how fast to push the drug. It is important to push the drug *slowly* over the required time period, monitoring the patient for any adverse reactions. It is also important to pace the delivery so half is pushed in over half the time. For example, if a drug is to be infused over 2 min, you should divide the volume and the time in half and count for 1 min, twice. Refer to a more detailed explanation of this in Chapter 10.

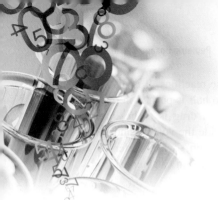

Complete the following problems:

1. The physician prescribed 10 mg of an antibiotic, PO, every 12 hr, for a 22-lb child. The safe dosage range is 0.5 to 2.0 mg/kg/day. The dosage range for this child is _____ mg per day. This is/ is not within a safe range. _____

2. The physician prescribed an antibiotic, 25 mg/kg for a 22-lb, 12-month-old child. The medicine was to be given q12h. The child should receive _____ mg per dose, every 12 hours.

3. A physician prescribed Phenergan for preoperative medication for a 44-lb child. Phenergan is to be given as 1 mg/kg of body weight. The nurse should give _____ mg preoperatively.

4. A physician prescribed Keflex 150 mg, PO, q6h. The child weighs 33 pounds. Keflex is labeled 125 mg per 5 mL. The safe dosage range is 25 to 50 mg/kg/day. The child's weight is _____ kg; the safe dosage range for this child per day is _____ mg. The child should receive _____ mL/q6h. This is/is not within a safe range. _____

5. A physician prescribed phenobarbital 50 mg, q12h, for a 66-lb child. The safe dosage range is 3 to 5 mg/kg/day. The child's weight is _____ kg; the safe dosage range for this child/day is _____ mg. The child should receive _____ mg/day. This is/is not within a safe range. _____

Critical Thinking Check

If the child gains 4 lb, would the dosage per day be within a safe range to give? _____ **Yes or No?**

---

6. A 10-year-old is ordered a stat dose of morphine sulfate IV for pain. The child weighs 90 lb and is 52 inches tall (4 feet, 4 inches). Calculate the dosage to administer using a BSA of 1.22 m². The normal adult dose of morphine sulfate is 10 mg. You should administer _____ mg of morphine sulfate. Morphine sulfate is available in 10 mg per 2 mL. You should administer _____ mL.

7. A physician prescribed a medication for a 7-year-old who weighs 70 lb and is 50 inches tall. The normal adult dose is 50 mg every 6 hr. Refer to the nomogram in Figure 14.1 to find the child's surface area in square meters. Determine the BSA: _____. Calculate the dosage the child should receive in four equally divided doses.

_____

8. The physician prescribed 20 mg of Demerol, every 6 hr postoperatively, to a 7-year-old child. Demerol is available as 25 mg per mL. You should give _____ mL/6 hr after verifying that the dose is safe.

9. The physician prescribed 5 mg of Garamycin for a child. The medication is available as 20 mg per 2 mL. To give 5 mg, you should give _____ mL.

10. The physician prescribed 325 mg of a suspension, PO, q12h, for a 44-kg child. The safe dosage is 15 mg/kg/day. The nurse would give _____ mg per day. Is this a safe dose? Yes ____ or No ____. The suspension is available as 500 mg per mL. The nurse would give ____ mL per dose.

11. The physician prescribed amoxicillin suspension 225 mg, PO, q8h, for a 33-lb child. The safe dosage range is 25 to 50 mg/kg/day. The safe dosage range for this child is _____ mg/day. Is this a safe dose? Yes _____ or No _____

12. The physician prescribed caffeine citrate 30 mg, PO, once a day for an 11-lb infant. The safe dosage range is 5 to 10 mg/kg/dose. Is this a safe dose? Yes ____ or No _____ .

13. The physician prescribed Ceclor 300 mg, PO, q8h, for a 66-lb child. The safe dosage range is 20 to 40 mg/kg/day. The safe dosage range for this child is _____ mg per day. Is this a safe dose? Yes ____ or No _____

14. The physician prescribed chloral hydrate 400 mg, PO, for one dose for an 11-lb infant prior to an EEG study. The safe dosage range is 25 to 50 mg/kg/dose. Is this a safe dose? Yes _____ or No _____

15. The physician prescribed Aldactone 20 mg, PO, q12h, for a 33-lb child. The safe dosage range is 1 to 3.3 mg/kg/24 hr. The safe dosage range for this child is _____ mg per dose. Is this a safe dose? Yes _____ or No _____

16. The physician prescribed Depakene 1 g, PO, q12h, for an 88-lb child. The safe dosage range is 30 to 60 mg/kg/day. The safe dosage range for this child is _____ mg per dose. The nurse would give _____ mg per dose. Is this a safe dose? Yes _____ or No _____

17. The physician prescribed Lasix 5 mg, PO, every morning, for an 11-lb infant with a cardiac problem. The safe dosage range is 0.5 to 2 mg/kg/day. The safe dosage range for this child is _____ mg per dose. Lasix liquid is labeled 10 mg per mL. The nurse would give _____ mL each morning. Is this a safe dose? Yes _____ or No _____

18. The physician prescribed gentamicin 12 mg, IV, q8h, for an infant who weighs 6 kg. The safe dosage is 2.5 mg/kg/dose. Gentamicin is available as 20 mg per mL. You would administer _____ mL, q8h. This is/is not a safe dose. _____

19. The physician prescribed morphine sulfate 5 mg, IV, q2h, p.r.n., for pain for a child who weighs 88 lb. The safe dosage range is 0.05 to 0.2 mg/kg/dose. Morphine sulfate is available as 15 mg per 1 mL. The child's weight is _____ kg; the safe dosage range for this child is _____ mg/dose. The child would receive _____ mL IV. This is/is not within a safe range. _____

20. The physician prescribed 300 mg of an antibiotic, IV, q6h, for a 66-lb child. The safe dosage range is 30 to 40 mg/kg/day. The child's weight is _____ kg; the safe dosage range for this child is _____. This child would receive _____ mg IV, q6h. This is/is not within a safe range. _____

21. The physician prescribed Lasix 40 mg, IV, stat, for an 88-lb child. The label reads, "Lasix, 10 mg per mL." The safe dosage range is 0.5 to 2 mg/kg/dose. The child's weight is _____ kg; the safe dosage range for this child is _____. This child would receive _____ mL. This is/is not within a safe range. _____

22. The physician prescribed ampicillin 250 mg in 30 mL of D5/0.22% NSS to infuse over 30 min, followed by a 15-mL flush. Ampicillin requires 5 mL for reconstitution. The drop factor is 60 gtt per mL. The pump or controller should be set at _____ mL per hr.

23. The physician prescribed Rocephin 500 mg in
50 mL of NSS to infuse over 30 min via a
Buretrol, followed by a 15-mL flush. Rocephin
requires 10 mL for reconstitution. The nurse
should set the controller at _____ mL per hr.

24. The physician prescribed gentamicin 10 mg in
50 mL of D5/0.45% NSS to infuse over 30 min
via a Buretrol, followed by a 15-mL flush. The
drop factor is 60 gtt per mL. Gentamicin is available as 20 mg per 2 mL. You should set the rate
at _____ mL per hr.

25. A child is to receive an IV medication of 75 mg
in 55 mL using NSS. The IV is to infuse over
45 min, followed by a 15-mL flush. A microdrip
Soluset is used. The nurse should set the pump at
_____ mL per hr.

26. A child is to receive Dilantin 25 mg per 2 mL in
10 mL using NSS. The IV is to infuse over
20 min via a microdrip Buretrol, followed by a
10-mL flush. The nurse should set the pump at
_____ mL per hr.

27. A child is to receive 1 g of an antibiotic. The
medication is to be diluted in 60 mL of D5/¼
NSS and to infuse over 30 min, followed by a
15-mL flush. It is a microdrop tubing. The
Buretrol is on a pump that should be set at
_____ mL per hr.

28. A child is to receive 30 mL of an intravenous solution every hour through a volume control set that delivers 60 microdrops per mL. The flow rate should be set at _____ gtt per min to deliver 30 mL/hr.

29. Give a child aminophylline 250 mg IVPB in 50 mL of NSS over 1 hr via a Buretrol that delivers 60 microdrops per mL, followed by a 10-mL flush. Aminophylline is available in 250 mg per 10 mL. You would give _____ gtt per min with a total volume of _____ mL.

30. The physician prescribed Solu-Medrol 20 mg by slow IV push for an asthmatic child. Solu-Medrol is labeled 40 mg per mL. The nurse should give _____ mL over 3 min.

31. An infant is to receive 15 mL of D5/0.22% NSS solution every hour through a volume control set that delivers 60 microdrops per mL. The flow rate should be set at _____ gtt per min to deliver 15 mL per hr.

---

thePoint. Additional practice problems to enhance learning and facilitate chapter comprehension can be found on **http://thePoint.lww.com/Boyer8e.**

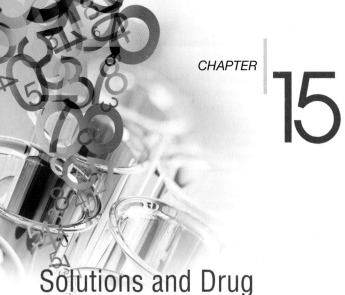

Solutions and Drug Reconstitution

LEARNING OBJECTIVES

After completing this chapter, you should be able to:

- Apply the basic steps for reconstituting medications packaged as powders.
- Calculate the reconstitution of an oral or enteral feeding.
- Calculate the preparation of a topical or irrigating solution.

Solutions are mixtures of liquids, solids, or gases (known as *solutes*) that are dissolved in a diluent (known as a *solvent*). Solutions can be administered externally (e.g., compresses, soaks, irrigations) or internally (e.g., parenteral medications, nutritional formulas).

Solutions can be prepared from full-strength drugs or from stock solutions. Full-strength drugs are considered to be 100% pure, whereas stock solutions contain drugs in a given solution strength, always less than 100%, from which weaker solutions are made. Solution strengths can be expressed in a percentage or ratio format; for example, a 1/2-strength solution means that there is one part solute to two parts total solution. *Remember:* the *less* solvent added, the *greater* is the solution strength; the *more* solvent added, the *weaker* is the solution strength.

Solution problems are basically problems involving percents that can be solved using the ratio and proportion method. When setting up the ratio and proportion for a solution made from a pure drug or from a stock solution, *use the strength of the desired solution to the strength of the available solution as one ratio, and the solute to the solution as the other ratio.*

desired solution strength : available solution strength
:: amount of solute : total amount of solution

You can substitute the Formula Method when using a proportion for a solution made from a stock solution:

$$\frac{\text{Desired strength}}{\text{Available strength}} \times \text{total amount of solution}$$

= amount of solute needed

$$\frac{D}{H} \times Q = x$$

When calculating solution problems, it is important to remember two things:

1. Work within the same measurement system (e.g., milligrams with milliliters, grains with minims).
2. Change solutions expressed in the fraction or colon format to a percent (1 : 2 or 1/2 is equal to 50%).

Reconstitution: Preparing Injections Packaged as Powders

Some medications are unstable in a liquid solution, so they are packaged as a powder. When the *available amount of a drug* is in a solute form (dry powder), the drug needs to be dissolved or reconstituted into a liquid form by adding a liquid diluent (solvent). The drug label, package insert, or reference material will list the manufacturer's directions for reconstitution (adding the diluent and mixing thoroughly). Although a pharmacist usually prepares the drug, a nurse may have to do so in some settings. Diluents for reconstitution must always be sterile when added to a dry powder. Sample diluents include:

- Bacteriostatic water
- Special packaged diluent
- Sodium chloride (0.9% NS) for injection
- Sterile water for injection

Reconstituted injectable medications are available in *single-strength* (either single- or multiple-dose vials) or *multiple-strength* solutions. *Remember:* For multiple-strength solutions, *the dosage strength depends on the amount of diluent*; for example, 75 mL of diluent may yield a solution of 200,000 units per mL, whereas 30 mL of diluent may yield 500,000 units per mL.

Basic Steps for Reconstitution

Remember: Always read the package insert or labeled directions for reconstitution very carefully because directions will vary for different medications. Follow these steps:

- Read the label for reconstitution directions.
- *Note* the length of time the medication will remain stable after reconstitution, preparation requirements (e.g., shake well), and storage requirements (e.g., temperature, protection from light).
- *Select* the type and quantity of recommended diluent.
- *Note* the total fluid volume. Reconstituted solutions will always exceed the volume of the added diluent. This added volume will determine the medication concentration (available dose).
- *Determine* the number of doses available in a multidose vial.
- *Label* the medication with the date and time of preparation, expiration, and reconstituted dosage if using a multiple-dose vial. *Note:* Some preparations allow for different quantities of diluent, which result in different solution strengths.
- *Initial* labeled vials.
- *Use* one of the three standard methods to calculate dosages.

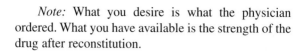

Note: What you desire is what the physician ordered. What you have available is the strength of the drug after reconstitution.

R U L E

To prepare a reconstituted medication: Follow the reconstitution directions (see previous steps), dilute powder, and withdraw prescribed dissolved fluid amount.

EXAMPLE #1:   Give 250 mg of Ancef, IM, every 8 hr. The medication is available as a powder in a 500-mg vial.

RECONSTITUTE: Labeled directions: Reconstitute by adding 2 mL of sterile water as a diluent. Shake well until dissolved. Solution concentration will equal 225 mg per mL. Total approximate available volume is 2.2 mL. Store at room temperature for 24 hr.

Ratio and Proportion

225 mg : 1 mL = 250 mg : x mL
225x = 250

$$x = \frac{\cancel{250}^{\,50}}{\cancel{225}_{\,45}} = \frac{50}{45} = 1.1 \text{ mL}$$

ANSWER: 1.1 mL

The Formula Method

$$\frac{D}{H} \times Q = x$$

$$\frac{250 \text{ mg}}{225 \text{ mg}} \times 1 \text{ mL}$$

$$\frac{\cancel{250}^{50}}{\cancel{225}_{45}} = \frac{50}{45} = 1.1 \text{ mL}$$

ANSWER: 1.1 mL

Dimensional Analysis

$$\frac{250 \text{ mg}}{225 \text{ mg}} \times \frac{1 \text{ mL}}{}$$

$$= \frac{250 \cancel{\text{ mg}}}{} \times \frac{1 \text{ mL}}{225 \cancel{\text{ mg}}} = \frac{250 \times 1 \text{ (mL)}}{225}$$

$$= \frac{\cancel{250}^{50}}{\cancel{225}_{45}} = \frac{50}{45} = 1.1 \text{ mL}$$

ANSWER: 1.1 mL

EXAMPLE #2: Give 125 mg of Solu-Medrol, IM. Medication is available as a powder in a 500-mg vial.

RECONSTITUTE: Labeled directions: Reconstitute by adding 8 mL of sterile water for injection. Solution concentration will equal 62.5 mg per mL. Total approximate available volume will be equal to or greater than 8 mL.

Ratio and Proportion

62.5 mg : 1 mL :: 125 mg : x mL
62.5x = 125

$$x = \frac{\cancel{125}^{2}}{\cancel{62.5}_{1}} = 2 \text{ mL}$$

ANSWER: 2 mL

The Formula Method

$$\frac{D}{H} \times Q = x$$

$$\frac{125}{62.5} \times 1 \text{ mL}$$

$$\frac{\cancel{125}^{2}}{\cancel{62.5}_{1}} = 2 \times 1 \text{ mL} = 2 \text{ mL}$$

ANSWER: 2 mL

Dimensional Analysis

$$\frac{125 \text{ mg}}{} \times \frac{1 \text{ mL}}{62.5 \text{ mg}}$$

$$= \frac{125 \ \cancel{\text{mg}}}{} \times \frac{1 \text{ mL}}{62.5 \ \cancel{\text{mg}}} = \frac{125 \times 1 \ (\text{mL})}{62.5}$$

$$= \frac{\cancel{125}^{2}}{\cancel{62.5}_{1}} = 2 \text{ mL}$$

ANSWER: 2 mL

Preparing an Oral or Enteral Feeding

When a person cannot eat, a tube can be placed in the stomach or duodenum (nasogastric tube) or inserted into the stomach (gastrostomy tube, PEG tube). Feedings, commercially prepared, are given as a bolus or via a feeding pump either intermittently or continuously (i.e., a Kangaroo pump). Sometimes the feeding solution needs to be prepared from a powder or diluted with sterile water or tap water. Refer to a nursing fundamentals textbook for review of the standard procedures for enteral feedings. See Figure 15.1.

R U L E

To prepare a specific strength solution from a given solution: Multiply the desired strength by the amount of solution (solute) and then subtract the solute from the total amount of solution (amount to be given).

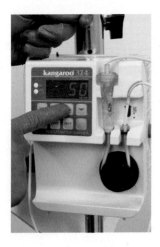

FIGURE 15.1 Enteral feeding pump. (From Taylor, C., Lillis, C., and LeMone, P. [2008]. *Fundamentals of nursing: The art and science of nursing care* [6th ed.]. Philadelphia: Lippincott Williams & Wilkins, page 1471.)

EXAMPLE #1:	Give 1/3-strength Sustacal every 6 hr through an NG tube. Sustacal is available in a 10-oz can (10 oz $\times$ 30 mL/oz = 300 mL).
MULTIPLY:	$1/3 \times 300$ mL = 100 mL (solute)
SUBTRACT:	300 mL – 100 mL = 200 mL (solvent to be dissolved).
ADD:	200 mL of water to 100 mL of Sustacal = 300 mL at 1/3 strength
GIVE:	300 mL over 6 hr. Set the feeding pump to 50 mL per hr.
FLUSH:	Flush tube with 50 mL. Monitor patient tolerance

> *ANSWER:* Give 300 mL over 6 hr. Set the feeding pump to 50 mL per hr.

EXAMPLE #2:	Give 1/2-strength Ensure 16 oz via a nasogastric tube q12h.
CONVERT:	16 oz = 480 mL (16 oz $\times$ 30 mL/oz)
MULTIPLY:	$1/2 \times 480$ mL = 240 mL (solute)
SUBTRACT:	480 mL – 240 mL (solvent to be dissolved)
ADD:	240 mL of water + 240 mL Ensure = 480 mL of 1/2-strength Ensure

> *ANSWER:* Give 480 mL over 12 hr. Set pump to 40 mL per hr. Flush tube with 50 mL.

Preparing a Topical Irrigating Solution

Preparing a Solution from a Solution

EXAMPLE #1: Prepare 1.0 liter (L) of a 10% solution from a pure drug.

The Formula Method

$$\frac{D}{H} \times Q = x$$

$$\frac{10\%}{100\%} = \frac{\overset{1}{10}}{100_{10}} = \frac{1}{10}$$

$$\frac{1}{10} \times 1{,}000 \text{ mL} = 100 \text{ mL}$$

ANSWER: 100 mL; measure 100 mL of pure drug and add 900 mL of water to prepare 1.0 L of a 10% solution.

EXAMPLE #2: Prepare 250 mL of a 5% solution from a 50% solution.

The Formula Method

$$\frac{D}{H} \times Q = x$$

$$\frac{5\%}{{}_1 50\%} \times \overset{5}{250} \text{ mL}$$

$$= 25 \text{ mL of solute needed}$$

ANSWER: The solution has a ratio strength of 1 : 10. Measure 25 mL of solute and add 225 mL of water to prepare 250 mL.

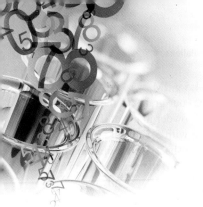

End of Chapter Review

Complete the following problems:

1. To prepare 400 mL of a 2% sodium bicarbonate solution from pure drug, you would need _____ g of solute.

2. To make 1.5 L of a 5% solution from a 25% solution, you would need _____ mL of solute. Add _____ mL of water to make 1.5 L.

3. There is 500 mL of 40% magnesium sulfate solution available for a soak. To make a 30% solution, you would need _____ mL of solute. Add _____ mL of water to make 500 mL.

4. The physician prescribed 500 mg of Cefizox, IM, every 12 hr, for a genitourinary infection. The medication is available as a powder in a 2-g vial. Reconstitute it with 6.0 mL of sterile water for injection and shake well. Solution concentration will provide 270 mg per mL. Fluid volume will equal 7.4 mL. Use approximate quantities for dosage calculations. Give _____ mL every 12 hr.

5. Methicillin sodium 1.5 g, IM, was prescribed for a systemic infection. Four grams of the medication is available as a powder in a vial. Directions state to reconstitute it with 5.7 mL of sterile water for injection and shake well. Solution concentration will provide 500 mg per mL. To give 1.5 g, the nurse should give _____ mL.

6. The physician prescribed 125 mg of Solu-Medrol, IM, for severe inflammation. The medication is available as a powder in a 0.5-g vial. Reconstitute it according to directions so that each 8 mL will contain 0.5 g of Solu-Medrol. The nurse would then give _____ mL to give 125 mg.

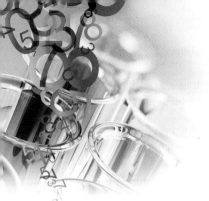

Solve the following drug administration problems and reduce each answer to its lowest terms.

1. Give 1.5 g. The drug is available in 250-mg tablets. Give _____ tablet(s).

2. Give 2 tsp. The drug is available as 250 mg per 5 mL. Give _____ mg.

3. Give 600 mg. The drug is available in 200-mg tablets. Give _____ tablet(s).

4. Give 0.3 g. The drug is available as 150 mg per 2.5 mL. Give _____ mL.

5. Give 75 mg. The drug is available as 25 mg per tsp. Give _____ mL.

Critical Thinking Check

Would it seem logical to give a tablespoon of medication to give 75 mg? _____ **Yes or No?**

---

6. Give 125 mg. The drug is available in 0.25-g tablets. Give _____ tablet(s).

7. Give gr 1/100. The drug is available in 0.6-mg tablets. Give _____ tablet(s).

8. Give 80 mg of a drug that is available as 240 mg per 3 mL. Give _____ mL.

9. Give 50 mg. The drug is available as 100 mg per 2 mL. Give _____ mL.

10. Give 0.75 mg. The drug is available as 500 mcg per 2 mL. Give _____ mL.

11. Give gr iii. The drug is available as 60 mg per mL. Give _____ mL.

12. Give gr 1/8. The drug is available as 15 mg per mL. Give _____ mL.

13. Give 0.3 mg. The drug is available as 200 mcg per mL. Give _____ mL.

14. Give gr 1/6. The drug is available as 8 mg per mL. Give _____ mL.

15. Give 0.25 g. The drug is available as 300 mg per 2 mL. Give _____ mL.

16. Give 500 mg of a medication that is available as a powder in a 2-g vial. Reconstitute it by adding 11.5 mL of sterile water for injection. Each 1.5 mL of solution contains 250 mg of the medication. Give _____ mL.

17. Give 1 g of a medication that is available as a powder in a 2-g vial. Reconstitute it by adding 5 mL to achieve a concentration of 330 mg per mL. Give _____ mL.

18. Give 125 mg of a drug dissolved in 100 mL of a solution over 30 min. You would give _____ mL per hr.

19. Give 1,000 mL of a solution over 8 hr, using a drop factor of 10 gtt per mL. Give _____ gtt per min.

Critical Thinking Check

If the available tubing had a drop factor of 15 gtt per mL, would you expect the gtt per min to be greater or less than the gtt per min for a drop factor of 10? _____ **Greater or Less than?**

20. Give 500 mL of a solution over 10 hr, using a drop factor of 60 gtt per mL. Give _____ gtt per min.

21. Give 1,000 mL of a solution over 6 hr, using a drop factor of 15 gtt per mL. Give _____ gtt per min.

22. Give 800 mL of a solution at 12 gtt per min, using a drop factor of 10 gtt per mL. Give over _____ hours and _____ minutes.

23. Give 250 mg of a solution in 500 mL at 10 mL per hr. Give _____ mg per hr.

24. Give 15 units of U-100 Regular insulin by subcutaneous injection. Use U-100 Regular insulin and
a U-100 syringe. Draw up insulin in the syringe
to the _____ -unit marking.

25. Give 35 units of NPH and 10 units of Regular
insulin, using U-100 insulin and U-100 syringes.
Draw up _____ units of _____ first, followed
by _____ units of _____.

26. Give 2,500 units of heparin subcutaneously.
Vial concentration is 5,000 units per mL.
Give _____ mL.

27. Give 1,000 mL of D5W with 15,000 units of
heparin to infuse at 30 mL per hr. Give _____
units per hr.

28. Give 1,000 mL of D5W with 40,000 units of
heparin to infuse at 25 mL per hr. Give _____
units per hr, which *is* or *is not* a safe dose. _____

29. An ER physician ordered 30 mg of a drug, IV,
stat, for a 154-lb teenager who had a tibia fracture.
The safe dosage range is 0.25 to 0.5 mg/kg/dose,
IV/IM. Is this a safe dose? Yes _____ or No _____

30. A physician prescribed 25 mg of a narcotic, IV,
q4h, as needed for pain for a 44-lb child. The safe
dosage range is 1 to 1.5 mg/kg/dose. The safe
dosage range for this child is _____ mg/dose.
The drug is available as 100 mg per 2 mL. The
nurse would give _____ mL. Is this a safe dose?
Yes _____ or No _____

31. A physician ordered Solu-Medrol 30 mg, IV, q12h, for an 88-lb child. The safe dosage range is 0.5 to 1.7 mg/kg/day. The safe dosage range for this child is _____ mg/day. Solu-Medrol is available as 40 mg per mL. The nurse would give _____ mL. Is this a safe dose? Yes _____ or No _____

32. The physician prescribed gentamicin 15 mg, IV, q8h, for a 6.5-kg infant. The safe dosage range is 6 to 7.5 mg/kg/day. The safe dosage range for this infant is _____ mg /day. Gentamicin is labeled 10 mg per mL for IV use. The nurse would give _____ mL. Is this a safe dose? Yes _____ or No _____

33. The physician prescribed vancomycin 0.4 g, IV, q8h, for a 66-lb child. The safe dosage is 40 mg/kg/day. The dosage range for this child is _____ mg per day. The nurse would give _____ mg q8h. Is this a safe dose? Yes _____ or No _____

34. The physician prescribed a narcotic 6 mg, IV, q3h, as needed for pain for a 110-lb child. The safe dosage range is 0.1 to 0.2 mg/kg/dose. The safe dosage range for this child is _____ mg/dose. Morphine is available as 15 mg per mL. The nurse would give _____ mL. Is this a safe dose? Yes _____ or No _____

35. The physician prescribed 1 mg, IM, of leucovorin calcium, to be given once a day for the treatment of megaloblastic anemia. The medication is available as a powder in a 50-mg

vial. Reconstitute it with 5.0 mL of bacteriostatic water for injection. Shake it well. Solution concentration will yield 10 mg per mL. Fluid volume will equal 5.0 mL. Give _____ mL, once a day.

36. The physician prescribed 25 mg of Librium, IM. Add 2 mL of special diluent to yield 100 mg per 2 mL. The nurse should give _____ mL.

Answer the next three questions by referring to the corresponding drug labels.

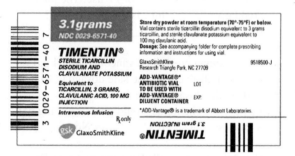

Timentin. (Courtesy of GlaxoSmithKline, Philadelphia, PA.)

37. The physician prescribed Timentin 3.1 g, IV, every 6 hr, for a patient with a severe infection. The patient would receive _____ g of Timentin in 24 hr.

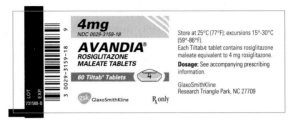

Avandia. (Courtesy of GlaxoSmithKline, Philadelphia, PA.)

38. The physician prescribed Avandia 8 mg twice a day. The patient would receive _____ mg in 24 hr.

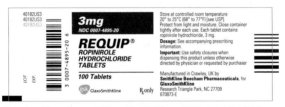

Requip. (Courtesy of GlaxoSmithKline, Philadelphia, PA.)

39. A patient with Parkinson's disease is to receive Requip, 3 mg, three times a day. The nurse would administer _____ tablet(s) each dose for a total of _____ mg in 24 hr.

40. In order to control a patient's blood glucose, an insulin infusion is prescribed. Insulin 100 units in 100 mL is started at 6 mL per hr. You document that the patient is receiving _____ units/hr.

41. Versed 50 mg in 100 mL is running at 3 mL per hr to manage anxiety in a mechanically ventilated patient. You document that the patient is receiving _____ mg per hr.

Answer the next two questions by referring to the corresponding drug label.

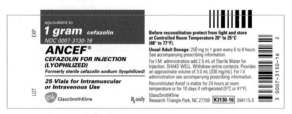

Ancef. (Courtesy of GlaxoSmithKline, Philadelphia, PA.)

42. A physician prescribed 1 g of Ancef, intramuscularly, every 8 hr. The nurse would need to mix _____ vial(s) for each dose.

43. A patient is prescribed 500 mg of Ancef intramuscularly, immediately. The nurse would reconstitute the vial of Ancef with _____ mL of sterile water for injection.

thePoint Additional practice problems to enhance learning and facilitate chapter comprehension can be found on **http://thePoint.lww.com/Boyer8e.**

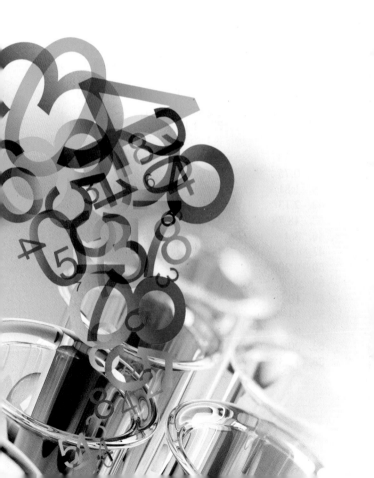

Answers

CHAPTER 1: Preassessment Test: Mathematics Skills Review

Basic Math Pretest: Pages 4–8

1. viii
2. xiii
3. x
4. xxxvii
5. Li
6. 15
7. 16
8. 65
9. 9
10. 19
11. 5/8
12. 1/2
13. 1/2
14. 4/15
15. 1/3
16. 1/150
17. 1/100
18. 3/4
19. 3/8
20. 8 2/5
21. 3/4
22. 6 1/8
23. 1/60
24. 3 3/7
25. 1/48
26. 2/5
27. 14/5
28. 27/4
29. 94/9
30. 57/7
31. 3
32. 4 1/18
33. 3 2/11
34. 1 3/13
35. 0.33
36. 0.40
37. 0.37
38. 0.75
39. 1.81
40. 4
41. 5.87
42. 2.13
43. 48.78
44. 0.250
45. 72
46. 3.4
47. 1/4
48. 4/5
49. 1/3
50. 9/20
51. 3/4
52. 3/5
53. 3
54. 16
55. 2.6
56. 10
57. 0.75
58. 12
59. 24
60. 0.16
61. 0.9
62. 0.2
63. 20%
64. 36%
65. 7%
66. 12.5%
67. 10.3%
68. 183%

69. 25%	70. 60%	71. 1%
72. 198%	73. 1.2%	74. 14.2%
75. 0.25	76. 0.4	77. 0.8
78. 0.15	79. 0.048	80. 0.0036
81. 0.0175	82. 0.083	
83. 18	84. 9	85. 1.08
86. 40	87. 25	88. 25%
89. 20%	90. 25%	91. 50
92. 120		

	Percent	Colon Ratio	Common Fractions	Decimal
93.	25%	25 : 100	1/4	0.25
94.	3.3%	1 : 30	1/30	0.033
95.	5%	5 : 100	1/20	0.05
96.	0.67%	1 : 150	1/150	0.0067
97.	0.45%	9 : 2,000	9/2,000	0.0045
98.	1%	1 : 100	1/100	0.01
99.	0.83%	1 : 120	1/120	0.0083
100.	50%	50 : 100	1/2	0.50

CHAPTER 2: Fractions
Practice Problems: Page 12

1. 7, 1/8, 7, 8	2. 9, 1/10, 10
3. 4, 1/5, 4, 5	4. 3, 1/4, 4

Practice Problems: Page 14

1. 1/2	2. 1/8	3. 1/9
4. 4/5	5. 4/6	6. 8/15

Order of size: smaller to larger value
1/300, 1/150, 1/100, 1/75, 1/25, 1/12, 1/9, 1/7, 1/3

Practice Problems: Pages 18–19

1. 12/20	2. 20/40	3. 2/4
4. 5/8	5. 3/5	6. 6/10
7. 1/6	8. 1/6	9. 1/4
10. 1/18		

Practice Problems: Page 20

1. 1/6	2. 1/6	3. 1/9
4. 1/6	5. 1/9	6. 1/4
7. 1/3	8. 3/5	

Practice Problems: Page 24

1. 69/12	2. 55/8	3. 43/5
4. 136/9	5. 98/3	6. 87/4
7. 37/2	8. 57/9	9. 27/5
10. 67/6		

Practice Problems: Pages 25–26

1. 7 1/2	2. 6 5/6	3. 7 5/9
4. 6 6/11	5. 7 1/2	6. 2 2/3
7. 4 3/10	8. 7 3/4	9. 9 5/9
10. 18 2/3		

Practice Problems: Pages 36–37

1. 2 5/11	2. 13/16	3. 3 19/24
4. 1 2/45	5. 1 3/10	6. 1 9/19
7. 1 3/14	8. 10 23/45	9. 1 5/8
10. 1 17/30	11. 3/7	12. 4/9
13. 13/30	14. 19/36	15. 5 16/21
16. 1 1/12		

Practice Problems: Pages 42–43

1. 16/45	2. 5/21	3. 3/20
4. 1 7/20	5. 21/32	6. 40/77
7. 6 3/4	8. 1 2/13	9. 1 5/9
10. 36	11. 29/50	12. 3 5/7

End of Chapter Review: Pages 44–46

1. 14/35, 15/35
2. 28/20, 4/20
3. 1/6
4. 1/8
5. 6 1/2
6. 13 1/8
7. 50/11
8. 209/23
9. 5/16
10. 1/8
11. 1/9
12. 5/28
13. 8/9
14. 1 1/3
15. 31/36
16. 7 5/24
17. 1/6
18. 5/9
19. 7/12
20. 4 9/40
21. 2 1/8
22. 11/24
23. 3/20
24. 3/11
25. 14
26. 8
27. 6/11
28. 10
29. 1 5/7
30. 24
31. 10 4/15
32. 5/56
33. 80
34. 4 1/2

CHAPTER 3: Decimals

Practice Problems: Pages 50–51

1. ten and one thousandths
2. three and seven ten-thousandths
3. eighty-three thousandths
4. one hundred and fifty-three thousandths
5. thirty-six and sixty-seven ten-thousandths
6. one hundred and twenty-five ten-thousandths
7. one hundred twenty-five and twenty-five thousandths
8. twenty and seventy-five thousandths
9. 5.037
10. 64.07
11. 0.020
12. 0.4
13. 8.064
14. 33.7
15. 0.015
16. 0.1

Practice Problems: Page 52

1. 0.75
2. 0.92
3. 1.75
4. 2.80

Practice Problems: Pages* 59–61

1. 38.2	2. 18.41	3. 84.64
4. 1.91	5. 19.91	6. 26.15
7. 243.58	8. 51.06	9. 12.33
10. 6.68	11. 66.25	12. 1.12
13. 22.51	14. 6.81	15. 101.4
16. 1065	17. 41.9	18. 7.94
19. 144.03	20. 400.14	21. 708.89
22. 30.54	23. 0.098	24. 0.0008
25. 9.32	26. 2.65	27. 10.89
28. 12.85		

Practice Problems: Pages* 64–65

1. 0.20	2. 0.125	3. 0.25
4. 0.067	5. 0.067	6. 0.053
7. 7/1,000	8. 93/100	9. 103/250
10. 5 3/100	11. 12 1/5	12. 1/8

End of Chapter Review: Pages* 66–68

1. five and four hundredths
2. ten and sixty-five hundredths
3. eight thousandths
4. eighteen and nineteenths

5. 6.08	6. 124.3	7. 16.001
8. 24.45	9. 59.262	10. 2.776
11. 5.21	12. 224.52	13. 0.128
14. 1.56	15. 5.35	16. 16.2
17. 6.77	18. 4.26	19. 8.47
20. 3,387.58	21. 0.77	22. 981.67
23. 0.33	24. 0.6	25. 0.143
26. 0.75	27. 9/20	28. 3/4
29. 3/50	30. 0.4	31. 0.22
32. 0.8	33. 6 4/5	34. 1 7/20
35. 8 1/2		

*See Appendix B: Answers have been rounded off.

CHAPTER 4: Percents, Ratio, and Proportion

Practice Problems: Page 74

1. 3/20
2. 3/10
3. 1/2
4. 3/4
5. 1/4
6. 3/5
7. 33 1/3%
8. 66.6%
9. 20%
10. 75%
11. 40%
12. 25%

Practice Problems: Page 78

1. 0.15
2. 0.25
3. 0.59
4. 0.80
5. 25%
6. 45%
7. 60%
8. 85%
9. 1/6 = 16.6%
10. 1/8 = 12.5%
11. 1/5 = 20%
12. 1/3 = 33.3%

Practice Problems: Pages 88–89

1. $\dfrac{50 \text{ mg}}{5 \text{ mL}}$; 50 mg : 5 mL; 50 mg/5 mL

2. $\dfrac{325 \text{ mg}}{1 \text{ tablet}}$; 325 mg : 1 tab; 325 mg/1 tab

3. $\dfrac{2 \text{ ampules}}{1 \text{ L}}$; 2 ampules : 1 L; 2 ampules/1 L

4. $\dfrac{250 \text{ mg}}{1 \text{ capsule}}$; 250 mg : 1 capsule; 250 mg/capsule

5. $\dfrac{1 \text{ tablet}}{5 \text{ grains}} = \dfrac{3 \text{ tablets}}{15 \text{ grains}}$

   1 tablet : 5 grains :: 3 tablets : 15 grains

6. $\dfrac{0.2 \text{ mg}}{1 \text{ tablet}} = \dfrac{0.4 \text{ mg}}{2 \text{ tablets}}$

   0.2 mg : 1 tablet :: 0.4 mg : 2 tablets

7. $\dfrac{10 \text{ mg}}{5 \text{ mL}} = \dfrac{30 \text{ mg}}{15 \text{ mL}}$

   10 mg : 5 mL = 30 mg : 15 mL

8. $x = 9$
9. $x = 18$

10. $x = 4$

11. $x = 50$

12. $\dfrac{50 \text{ mg}}{1 \text{ mL}} = \dfrac{40}{x \text{ mL}}$

　　$50x = 40 \qquad x = 0.8 \text{ mL}$

13. $\dfrac{25 \text{ mg}}{1 \text{ mL}} = \dfrac{x \text{ mg}}{1.5 \text{ mL}}$

　　$x = 25 \times 1.5 \qquad x = 37.5 \text{ mg}$

14. $\dfrac{0.125 \text{ mg}}{1 \text{ tablet}} = \dfrac{x}{2 \text{ tablets}}$

　　$x = 0.125 \times 2 \qquad x = 0.25 \text{ mg}$

15. $1 \text{ g}/5 \text{ mL} = x \text{ g}/15 \text{ mL}$

　　$5x = 15 \qquad x = 3 \text{ g}$

End of Chapter Review: Pages 90–94

	Percent	Fraction	Decimal
1.	16.6%	1/6	0.166
2.	25%	1/4	0.25
3.	6.4%	8/125	0.064
4.	21%	21/100	0.21
5.	40%	2/5	0.40
6.	162%	1 31/50	1.62
7.	27%	27/100	0.27
8.	5 1/4%	21/400	0.052
9.	450%	9/2	4.50
10.	8 1/3%	1/12	0.083
11.	1%	1/100	0.01
12.	85.7%	6/7	0.857
13.	450%	18/4	4.5
14.	150%	1 1/2	1.5
15.	72%	18/25	0.72

16. $\dfrac{10 \text{ mg}}{1 \text{ tablet}}$; 10 mg : 1 tab

17. $\dfrac{10 \text{ units}}{1 \text{ mL}}$; 10 units : 1 mL

18. $\dfrac{200 \text{ mg}}{1 \text{ kg}}$; 200 mg : kg

19. $\dfrac{100 \text{ mg}}{1 \text{ tablet}} = \dfrac{300 \text{ mg}}{x \text{ tablets}}$

    100 mg : 1 tablet :: 300 mg : x tablets

20. $\dfrac{250 \text{ mg}}{1 \text{ tablet}} = \dfrac{500 \text{ mg}}{x \text{ tablets}}$

    250 mg : 1 tablet :: 500 mg : x tablets

21. $\dfrac{0.075 \text{ mg}}{1 \text{ tablet}} = \dfrac{0.15 \text{ mg}}{x \text{ tablets}}$

    0.075 mg : 1 tablet :: 0.15 mg : x tablet

22. $\dfrac{250 \text{ mg}}{0.5 \text{ mL}} = \dfrac{500 \text{ mg}}{x \text{ mL}}$

    250 mg : 0.5 mL :: 500 mg : x mL

23. $\dfrac{4}{5}$ or 0.8

24. 6

25. 4.5

26. $x = 6$

27. 20 mg : 1 mL :: 10 mg : x mL

    20 mg $\times$ x mL = 10 mg $\times$ 1 mL

    $20x = 10$

    $\dfrac{\cancel{20}^{1} x}{\cancel{20}_{1}} = \dfrac{\cancel{10}^{1}}{\cancel{20}_{2}} = \dfrac{1}{2}$ mL

    Answer: $\dfrac{1}{2}$ mL

Verify the Answer:

EXTREMES

20 mg : 1 mL :: 10 mg : $\frac{1}{2}$(0.5) mL

MEANS

20 mg × 0.5 mL = 10 mg × 1 mL

$20 \times 0.5 = 10$ ⎤ Sum products
$10 \times 1 = 10$ ⎦ are equal

CTC* = Yes

28. $\dfrac{50 \text{ mg}}{5 \text{ mL}} = \dfrac{25 \text{ mg}}{x \text{ mL}}$

Cross-multiply:
50 mg × x mL = 25 mg × 5 mL
$50x = 125$

$\dfrac{\overset{1}{\cancel{50}}x}{\cancel{50}_1} = \dfrac{\overset{5}{\cancel{125}}}{\cancel{50}_2}$

$x = \dfrac{5}{2} = 2\dfrac{1}{2}$ mL

ANSWER: 2.5 mL

Verify the Answer:

$\dfrac{50 \text{ mg}}{5 \text{ mL}} = \dfrac{25 \text{ mg}}{2.5 \text{ mL}}$

$50 \times 2.5 = 125$ ⎤ Sum products
$25 \times 5 = 125$ ⎦ are equal

CTC = Yes

*CTC = Critical Thinking Check

29. $3.0 \text{ mg} : 1.0 \text{ mL} :: 1.5 \text{ mg} : x \text{ mL}$

$3.0 \text{ mg} \times x \text{ mL} = 1.5 \text{ mg} \times 1.0 \text{ mL}$

$3x = 1.5$

$$\frac{\cancel{3}^{1}x}{\cancel{3}_{1}} = \frac{\cancel{1.5}^{1}}{\cancel{3}_{2}} = \frac{1}{2}$$

$$x = \frac{1}{2} \text{ mL}$$

ANSWER: $\frac{1}{2}$ mL

Verify the Answer:

┌──────EXTREMES──────┐
$3.0 \text{ mg} : 1.0 \text{ mL} :: 1.5 \text{ mg} : 0.5 \text{ mL}$
　　　　　└─MEANS─┘

$3.0 \text{ mg} \times 0.5 \text{ mL} = 1.5 \text{ mg} \times 1.0 \text{ mL}$

$\left.\begin{array}{l} 3.0 \times 0.5 = 1.5 \\ 1.5 \times 1.0 = 1.5 \end{array}\right\}$ Sum products are equal

CTC = Yes

30. $20 \text{ mg} : 2 \text{ mL} :: 25 \text{ mg} : x \text{ mL}$

$20 \text{ mg} \times x \text{ mL} = 25 \text{ mg} \times 2 \text{ mL}$

$20x = 50$

$$\frac{^{1}\cancel{20}}{^{1}\cancel{20}} = \frac{^{5}\cancel{50}}{^{2}\cancel{20}} = \frac{5}{2} = 2.5 \text{ mL}$$

ANSWER: 2.5 mL

Verify the Answer:

$20 \text{ mg} : 2 \text{ mL} = 25 \text{ mg} : 2.5 \text{ mL}$

$20 \text{ mg} \times 2.5 \text{ mL} = 25 \text{ mg} \times 2 \text{ mL}$

$\left.\begin{array}{l} 20 \times 2.5 = 50 \\ 25 \times 2 = 50 \end{array}\right\}$ Sum products are equal

CTC = Yes

31. 7.5 mL
32. 7.5 mL
33. 0.5 mL
34. 1.5 mL
35. 1.6 mL
36. 0.7 mL
37. 3 tablets

End of Unit 1 Review: Pages 95–97

1.	1	2.	1/15
3.	7/10	4.	5/12
5.	4/15	6.	1/16
7.	1/75	8.	1/150
9.	2	10.	4/5
11.	1/4	12.	3 1/3
13.	1/3	14.	1/6
15.	1/100	16.	5/30
17.	3.1	18.	4.26
19.	0.4	20.	5.68
21.	2.5	22.	15
23.	16.67	24.	1.89
25.	0.8	26.	0.25
27.	0.33	28.	1/2
29.	7/100	30.	1 1/2
31.	1/4	32.	1/300
33.	3/500	34.	40%
35.	450%	36.	2%

37. 12 (4 × 12 & 3 × 16 = 48)
38. 1 1/5 (25 × 1.2 & 20 × 1.5 = 30)
39. 1 1/4 (8 × 1.2 & 1 × 10 = 10)
40. 1 3/5 (4/5 × 50 & 25 × 1.6 = 40)
41. 1/2 (500 × 1/2 & 1,000 × 1/4 = 250)
42. 0.5 (100 × 1/2 & 2 × 2.5 = 50)

43.	180	44.	2
45.	1/9	46.	600
47.	1 3/5	48.	5
49.	3 1/3	50.	90
51.	1	52.	1/4
53.	1.87	54.	2
55.	1		

CHAPTER 5: The Metric, Household, and Apothecary Systems of Measurement

Practice Problems: Pages 113–114

1.	0.036 m	2.	41.6 dm
3.	0.08 cm	4.	0.002 m
5.	2.05 cm	6.	180 mm
7.	3,000 mm	8.	0.02 m
9.	60 mm	10.	1 m
11.	0.0036 L	12.	61.7 mL
13.	900 mL	14.	64 mg
15.	1.0 g	16.	0.008 dg
17.	800 cg	18.	1,600 mL
19.	0.0416 L	20.	3,200 mg

End of Chapter Review: Pages 118–120

1.	0.00743 m	2.	0.006 dm
3.	10,000 m	4.	6,217 mm
5.	0.0164 dL	6.	0.047 L
7.	1,000 cL	8.	569 mL
9.	0.0356 g	10.	30 cg
11.	50 mg	12.	930 mg
13.	0.1 mg	14.	2,000 mcg
15.	0.001 mg	16.	7,000 g
17.	4,000 mcg	18.	13,000 g
19.	2,500 mL	20.	600 mcg
21.	80 mg	22.	10 mcg

23. 0.06 g
24. 10,500 mcg
25. 0.0005 L
26. 1 dg
27. 0.35 g
28. 0.0034 g
29. 30,000 mcg
30. 0.13 g
31. 2,000 g
32. 18,000 mL
33. 450,000 mg
34. 0.04 mg
35. 80 dL
36. 1,000 cL
37. 460 dg
38. 500 mg
39. 0.5 L
40. 25,000 g
41. gr iii
42. drams v
43. gr v
44. mx
45. mxxss̅
46. pt v
47. 2 gal
48. ½ oz
49. 1 oz
50. 2 g
51. 2 qt
52. ¼ pt
53. 4 drams
54. 2 teacups
55. 24 oz
56. 3 oz
57. 120 gtt
58. 9 tsp
59. 16 oz
60. ½ pt

CHAPTER 6: Approximate Equivalents and System Conversions
Practice Problems: Pages 125–126

1. 360 mL
2. 0.0003 L
3. 2 tbsp
4. 0.75 gr
5. 10 mL
6. 66 lb
7. 0.3 mg
8. 1,500 mL
9. 2 g
10. 0.3 mg
11. 1 oz
12. 60 mL
13. 1/10 gr
14. 45 gr
15. 1 qt
16. 2 L
17. 1 kg
18. 15 mL

End of Chapter Review: Pages 127–129

1. 25 kg
2. 30 gr
3. 960 mL per day
4. 4 inches
5. 2 tsp
6. 300 to 325 mg
7. 3 gtt
8. 1/150 gr

9. 1-ounce
10. 18 kg; 180 mg
11. 1.8 g
12. 2 ounces
13. 6 tablets
14. 1 tsp
15. 0.4 g
16. 250 mg; 1 g
17. 450 mL
18. 2 tsp
19. 1 tbsp
20. 2 tablets; 0.6 mg

End of Unit 2 Review: Pages 130–131

1. 80 mg
2. 3,200 mL
3. 1.5 mg
4. 125 mcg
5. 20,000 g
6. 0.005 g
7. 70 kg
8. 30 gtt
9. 1 g
10. 16 ounces
11. 1 1/2 qt
12. 1 ounce
13. 3 tsp
14. 1 ounce
15. 6 ounces
16. 1 ounce
17. 30 mg
18. 1 ounce
19. 30 mL
20. 60 to 65 mg
21. 15 mL
22. 44 lb
23. 0.4 mg
24. 1/200 gr
25. 54 mL
26. 4 tsp
27. 8,500 mg
28. 0.95 g
29. 1/4 gr
30. 6,000 mcg

CHAPTER 7: Medication Labels
Practice Problems: Pages 141–143
FIGURE 7.2 (Augmentin)

1. Amoxicillin/clavulanate potassium
2. 200 mg per 5 mL
3. Keep tightly closed. Shake well before using. Must be refrigerated. Discard after 10 days.
4. Add 2/3 of total water for reconstitution.
5. Each 5 mL contains amoxicillin 200 mg.
6. 50 mL.

FIGURE 7.3 (Ancef)

1. Cefazolin
2. Intramuscular and intravenous
3. Add 2.5 mL of sterile water for injection
4. 330 mg/mL (IM use)
5. 250 mg to 1 g, every 6 hr to 8 hr
6. Shake well. Before reconstitution, protect from light and store at 20 to 25 degrees Celsius (room temperature).

FIGURE 7.4 (Requip)

1. Ropinirole hydrochloride
2. NDC 0007—4895-20
3. 3 mg
4. 100 tablets
5. Tablets
6. Protect from light and moisture. Close container tightly after each use.
7. Requip
8. GlaxoSmithKline

End of Chapter Review: Pages 144–146
FIGURES 7.5 to 7.8 (Tagamet, Amoxil, Augmentin, Paxil)

1. 2 tablets; 1,200 mg
2. 500 mg; 1 tablet
3. 2.5 mL; 300 mg; 7.5 mL
4. 1 tablet; 80 mg

CHAPTER 8: Oral Dosage Calculations
Practice Problems: Pages 166–168

1. 4 tablets
2. 15 mL
3. 1/2 tablet
4. 10 mL
5. 3 tablets
6. 2 tablets
7. 5 mL
8. 1/2 tablet
9. 2 tablets; CTC = No
10. 10 mL; CTC = No

11. 15 mL; 30 mg   12. ½ tsp; 7.5 mL
13. 1 mg
14. 2 mL   15. 4 mL
16. 4 tablets   17. 0.6 mL
18. 0.3 mL   19. 3 tablets
20. 2½ tablets

End of Chapter Review: Pages 169–171

1. 3 tablets   2. 3 tablets
3. 30 mL   4. 4 tablets
5. 1 tablet   6. 2 tablets
7. 1 ounce   8. 1 tablet
9. 7.5 mL   10. 1 tablet
11. 1 tablet; 4 tablets   12. 4 tablets
13. 2 tsp: 14. 500 mg
15. 4 tablets   16. 4 tablets; CTC = Yes
17. 10 mL; 2 tsp;
    CTC = Yes

CHAPTER 9: Parenteral Dosage Calculations
End of Chapter Review: Pages 186–190

1. 2 mL   2. 2 mL
3. 3 mL   4. 2 mL
5. 0.8 mL
6. 0.4 mL   7. 0.75 mL
8. 0.7 mL   9. 3 mL
10 0.6 mL   11. 0.25 mL
12. 0.75 mL   13. 1.25 mL
14. 0.8 mL   15. 0.8 mL; CTC = No
16. 0.6 mL   17. 0.75 mL
18. 0.5 mL   19. 2 mL
20. 2 mL   21. 0.5 mL
22. 1.5 mL   23. 1 mL
24. 2 mL   25. 0.5 mL

26.	1.5 mL	27.	2.5 mL
28.	4 mL	29.	1 mL
30.	1.2 mL	31.	0.5 mL
32.	0.5 mL	33.	4 mL; CTC = No. Limit injection to 3 mL per site.

CHAPTER 10: Intravenous Therapy
Practice Problems: Pages 213–215

1. 83 mL per hr; CTC = Yes
2. 125 mL per hr
3. 27 gtt per min
4. 42 gtt per min
5. 21 gtt per min
6. 17 gtt per min; CTC = slower at 15 gtt per min
7. 17 gtt per min
8. 19 gtt per min
9. 17 gtt per min
10. 50 gtt per min
11. 19 gtt per min
12. 17 gtt per min
13. 25 mL; 25 gtt per min; CTC = Yes
14. 67 gtt per min

End of Chapter Review: Pages 216–218

1. 63 mL per hr
2. 100 mL per hr
3. 250 mL per hr
4. 83 mL per hr
5. 50 mL per hr
6. 63 mL per hr
7. 21 gtt per min
8. 42 gtt per min
9. 167 mL per hr; 28 gtt per min
10. 10 gtt per min
11. 19 gtt per min
12. 8 gtt per min
13. 20 hr
14. 12½ hr
15. 12½ hr
16. 13 gtt per min
17. 42 gtt per min
18. 38 gtt per min
19. 100 gtt per min
20. 125 mL

CHAPTER 11: Intravenous Therapies: Critical Care Applications
End of Chapter Review: Pages 233–237

1. 3 mL per hr; CTC = Yes
2. 4 mg per min
3. 15.2 mL per hr; CTC = decrease
4. 22.2 mcg/kg/min
5. 3 mL per hr
6. 40 mL; 1 mg per mL; 60 mL per hr
7. 1 mL; 200 mL per hr; 24 mL per hr
8. 2 mL; 25 mL per hr; 10 mL per hr
9. 7.2 mcg/kg/min; CTC = Increase
10. 7.5 mL per hr; 80 mcg per min
11. 10 mL per hr
12. 200 mcg per mL; 68.2 mL per hr
13. 10 mL; 6 mL per hr
14. 11.2 mL per hr; CTC = Increase; Decrease
15. 6 mL per hr
16. 4 mcg per min
17. 10 mL per hr
18. 14.2 mL per hr

CHAPTER 12: Insulin
End of Chapter Review: Pages 254–257

1. 60 units of U-100

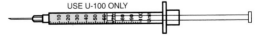

2. 82 units of U-100

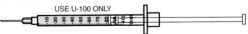

3. 45 units of U-50

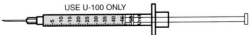

4. 35 units of U-50

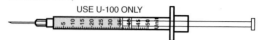
USE U-100 ONLY

5. 26 units of U-50

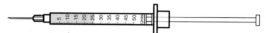

6. 56 units of U-100

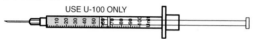
USE U-100 ONLY

7. 60 units
8. 40 units
9. 20 units
10. 70 units
11. 21; U-50/0.5 mL
12. 45; U-50/0.5 mL
13. 64; U-100/1 mL
14. 38; U-50/0.5 mL
15. 30; U-50/0.5 mL
16. U-50; 30 units;
    CTC = Not Logical
17. 39 units; U-50
18. 15 units
19. 50 units; CTC = Yes
20. 34 units; NPH

CHAPTER 13: Heparin Preparation and Dosage Calculations: Subcutaneous and Intravenous
End of Chapter Review: Pages 276–279

1. 400 units per hr; safe
2. Yes
3. 20 mL per hr
4. 4,480 units; 20.2 mL per hr
5. 22.4 mL per hr; CTC = Less Than
6. 11.4 units/kg/hr
7. 0.6 mL; 20,000 units; is within
8. 0.8 mL; 24,000 units; is within;
   CTC = 15,000 units per 8 hr
9. 0.6 mL; 10,000 units; is within
10. 0.25 mL
11. 600 units per hr

12. 45,000; unsafe
13. 50 mL per hr
14. 21 mL per hr; 625 units per hr
15. 12.7 mL per hr
16. 13.1 units/kg/hr

CHAPTER 14: Pediatric Dosage Calculations and Intravenous Therapy

Practice Problems: Pages 297–300

1. No; safe dosage range is 300 mg per day
2. Yes; safe dosage range is 100 to 200 mg per day
3. 4 mg; Yes; safe dosage range is 0.8 to 4 mg per dose
4. 11 mL
5. 40 kg; 50 to 70 mg per dose; Yes
6. 60 kg; 3 to 6 g per day; Yes
7. 30 kg; 750 to 1,500 mg per day; Yes
8. 15 kg; 75 to 150 mg per day; Yes
9. 20 kg; 10 to 20 mg per day; 4 mL; Yes
10. 25 to 50 mg per day; Yes
11. 25 to 100 mg per day; Yes
12. 80 to 120 mg per dose; 1 mL; Yes
13. 300 mg to 600 mg per day; Yes; CTC = No, 24-hr total = 900 mg
14. 1.5 mL
15. BSA = 0.7 m^2; 260 mg; 2.6 mL

End of Chapter Review: Pages 310–316

1. 5 to 20 mg per day; is safe
2. 250 mg
3. 20 mg
4. 15 kg; 375 to 750 mg; 6 mL per q6h = 600 mg per day; is safe
5. 30 kg; 90 to 150 mg per day; 100 mg; is safe; CTC = Yes

6. 7 mg; 1.4 mL
7. BSA = 1.10 m^2; dosage = 31.5-mg dose
8. 0.8 mL
9. 0.5 mL
10. 650 mg per day; Yes; 0.65 mL
11. 375 to 750 mg per day; Yes
12. Yes
13. 600 to 1,200 mg per day; Yes
14. No
15. 7.5 to 24.75 mg per dose; Yes
16. 600 to 1,200 mg per dose; 1,000 mg; Yes
17. 2.5 to 10 mg per day; 0.5 mL; Yes
18. 0.6 mL; is safe
19. 40 kg; 2 to 8 mg per dose; 0.33 mL; is safe
20. 30 kg; 9,00 to 1,200 mg per day; 300 mg; is safe
21. 40 kg; 20 to 80 mg per dose; 4 mL; is safe
22. 100 mL per hr
23. 150 mL per hr
24. 100 mL per hr
25. 93 mL per hr
26. 60 mL per hr
27. 150 mL per hr
28. 30 gtt per min
29. 60 gtt per min; 60 mL
30. 0.5 mL
31. 15 gtt per min

CHAPTER 15: Solutions and Drug Reconstitution
End of Chapter Review: Pages 327–328

1. 8 g
2. 300 mL; 1,200 mL
3. 375 mL; 125 mL
4. 1.85 or 1.9 mL
5. 3 mL
6. 2 mL

End of Unit 3 Review: Pages 329–336

1. 6 tablets
2. 500 mg
3. 3 tablets
4. 5 mL
5. 15 mL; CTC = Yes
6. 1/2 tablet
7. 1 tablet
8. 1 mL
9. 1 mL
10. 3 mL
11. 3 mL
12. 0.5 mL
13. 1.5 mL
14. 1.25 mL
15. 1.7 mL
16. 3 mL
17. 3 mL
18. 200 mL
19. 21 gtt per min; CTC = Greater at 32 gtt/min
20. 50 gtt per min (approximate)
21. 42 gtt per min (approximate)
22. 11 hr; 6 min
23. 5 mg/hr
24. 15-unit
25. 10 units of Regular; 35 units of NPH
26. 0.5 mL
27. 450 units per hr
28. 1,000 units per hr; is a safe dose
29. Yes
30. 20 to 30 mg per dose; 0.5 mL; Yes
31. 20 to 68 mg per day; 0.75 mL; Yes
32. 39 to 48.75 mg per day; 1.5 mL; Yes
33. 1,200 mg per day; 400 mg; Yes
34. 5 to 10 mg per dose; 0.4 mL; Yes
35. 0.1 mL
36. 0.5 mL
37. 12.4 g
38. 16 mg
39. 1 tablet; 9 mg
40. 6 units/hr
41. 1.5 mg/hr
42. 1 vial
43. 2.5 mL

Appendix B: Rounding Off Decimals
Practice Problems: Page 365

1. 0.8	2. 0.3
3. 0.2	4. 1.2
5. 2.7	6. 3.8

1. 0.55	2. 0.74
3. 1.68	4. 1.23
5. 2.47	6. 4.38

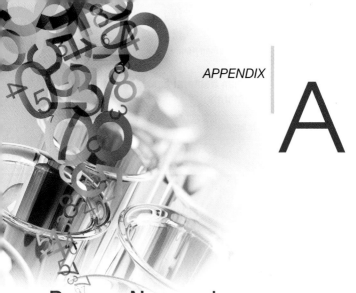

Roman Numerals

The use of Roman numerals dates back to ancient times when symbols were used for pharmaceutical computations and record keeping. Modern medicine still uses Roman numerals in prescribing medications, especially when using the apothecary system of weights and measurement.

The Roman system uses letters to designate numbers; the most commonly used letters are shown in Table A-1. Lowercase Roman numerals are used to express numbers. The most common letters you will use are one (i), five (v), and 10 (x). Four numerals are rarely used in practice (50, 100, 500, 1,000) but are included in the table.

The Roman numeral system follows certain rules for arrangement of its numerals.

RULE

To read and write Roman numerals, follow these steps:

Table A.1 **Roman Numeral Equivalents for Arabic Numerals**

ARABIC NUMERAL	ROMAN NUMERAL
1	i
2	ii
3	iii
4	iv
5	v
6	vi
7	vii
8	viii
9	ix
10	x
20	xx
40	xL
50	L
100	C

- Add values when the *largest* valued numeral is on the *left* and the *smallest* valued numeral is on the *right*.

EXAMPLES: xv = 10 + 5 = 15
            xxv = 20 + 5 = 25

- Subtract values when the *smallest*-valued numeral is on the *left* and the *largest*-valued numeral is on the *right*.

EXAMPLES: ix = 10 − 1 = 9
            iv = 5 − 1 = 4

- *Subtract* values *first* and then *add* when the *smallest-*valued numeral is in the *middle* and the *larger* values are on either side.

EXAMPLES: xiv = (5 − 1) + 10 = 4 + 10 = 14
             xix = (10 − 1) + 10 = 9 + 10 = 19

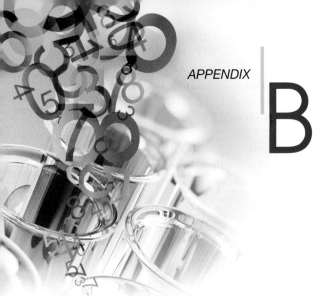

Rounding Off Decimals

To round off decimals, follow these steps:

- Determine the place that the decimal is to be "rounded off" to (tenths, hundredths). For example, let's round off 36.315 to the nearest hundredth.
- Bracket the number [ ] in the hundredths place (2 places to the right of the decimal). For 36.315, you would bracket the 1. Then 36.315 would look like this: 36.3[1]5.
- Look at the number to the right of the bracket. For 36.3[1]5, that number would be 5.
- If the number to the right of the bracket is less than 5 (<5), then drop the number. If it is 5 or greater than 5 (>5), then increase the bracketed number by 1.

For 36.3[1]5, increase the bracketed number [1] by 1. The rounded off number becomes 36.32.

EXAMPLE:

5.671
5.6[7]1
Look at the number to the right of [7].
The number is <5.
Leave [7] as is; drop 1.
[7] stays as [7].
5.671 rounds off to 5.67.

ANSWER: 5.67

PRACTICE PROBLEMS

Round off to the nearest tenth.

1. 0.83 _____   2. 0.34 _____

3. 0.19 _____   4. 1.19 _____

5. 2.66 _____   6. 3.84 _____

Round off to the nearest hundredth.

1. 0.545 _____   2. 0.737 _____

3. 1.680 _____   4. 1.231 _____

5. 2.468 _____   6. 4.383 _____

Answers are on p. 360.

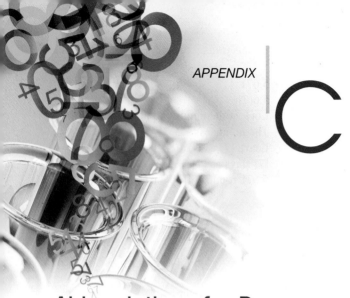

Abbreviations for Drug Preparation and Administration

The Institute for Safe Medication Practices (ISMP) has compiled a list of frequently misinterpreted abbreviations that can cause medication errors. The complete list can be found at http://www.ismp.org. Some abbreviations frequently used in the past are no longer acceptable. The correct approach is to write the word out in full.

ABBREVIATION	INTERPRETATION
a or ā	before
@*	Use "at"
aa or āā	of each
a.c.	before meals
A.D.*	Use "right ear"

*Do not use, per ISMP recommendations.

ABBREVIATION	INTERPRETATION
ad lib.	as desired
A.L. or A.S.*	Use "left ear"
alt. h.	alternate hour
AM	before noon
aq.	water
A.S.A.P.	as soon as possible
A.U.*	Use "each ear"
b.i.d.	twice a day
b.i.n.	twice a night
b.i.w.	twice a week
c̄	with
C	gallon
cap(s).	capsule(s)
CD	controlled dose
cm	centimeter
CR	controlled release
D/C*	Use "discontinue"
DS	double strength
dil.	dilute
disp.	dispense
dr	Use "dram"
Dx	diagnose
elix.	elixir
ext.	extract; external
g	gram
gal	gallon
gr	grain
gtt	drops
h, hr	hour
Ⓗ	hypodermic
h.s.	hour of sleep; at bedtime
ID	intradermal
IM	intramuscular
IN	intranasal
IV	intravenous
IVPB	intravenous piggyback
kg	kilogram
KVO	keep vein open

*Do not use, per ISMP recommendations.

ABBREVIATION	INTERPRETATION
L	liter
LA	long acting
lb	pound
M; m	meter
m; min	minim
mcg	microgram
mEq	milliequivalent
mg	milligram
mL	milliliter
mm	millimeter
NGT	nasogastric tube
noct., NOC	at night
N.P.O.	nothing by mouth
NS	normal saline solution
O.	pint
O.D.*	Use "right eye"
o.d.; q.d.	once every day
o.h.	every hour
oint	ointment
o.m.	every morning
o.n.	every night
O.S.*	Use "left eye"
OTC	over-the-counter
O.U.*	Use "each eye"
oz	ounce
$\bar{p}$	after
p.c.	after meals
per	by
p.o. or per os*	Use "by mouth" or "orally"
PM	evening, before midnight
p.r.n.	as needed; when necessary
pt	pint
q*	Use "each," "every"
q.a.m.	every morning
qh	every hour
q.i.d.	four times a day
q2h	every 2 hours
q3h	every 3 hours

*Do not use, per ISMP recommendations.

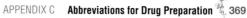

ABBREVIATION	INTERPRETATION
q4h	every 4 hours
q6h	every 6 hours
q8h	every 8 hours
q12h	every 12 hours
q.o.d.*	Use "every other day"
q.s.	quantity sufficient; as much as needed
qt	quart
R, rect	rectally
R$_x$	to take; by prescription
R/O	rule out
$\bar{s}$	without
$\overline{ss}$*	Use "one-half" or "½"
SC, s.c.; s.q., sub q	Use "subcutaneously" or "subcut"
sig.	label; write
SL; subl.	sublingual
sol; soln	solution
s.o.s.	one dose as necessary
SR	sustained release
stat.	immediately
supp.	suppository
susp.	suspension
tab	tablet
tbsp	tablespoon
t.i.d.	three times a day
tinct; tr	tincture
T.K.O.	to keep open
tsp; t	teaspoon
ung.	ointment
vag.	vaginally
XL	long acting
XR	extended release

*Do not use, per ISMP recommendations.

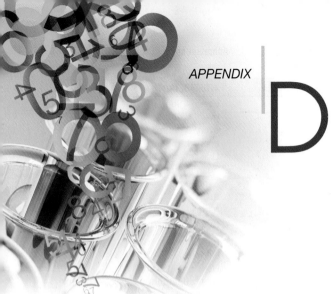

Intradermal Injections

The *intradermal route* is preferred for:

- Small quantities of medication (0.1 mL to 0.2 mL)
- Nonirritating solutions that are slowly absorbed
- Allergy testing and local anesthesia for invasive tests
- PPD administration (screening for tuberculosis)

Note: A raised or reddened area indicates a positive reaction

The Intradermal Route

Use
A tuberculin syringe

Inject about 1/8 inch
Into dermis under the outer layer of skin or epidermis. Make sure the bevel of the needle is up. Inject slowly until the solution creates a small wheal (blister).

The Intradermal Route (continued)

Angle
15 degrees

15°↑

Site
Inner surface of forearm

Administering an Intradermal Injection

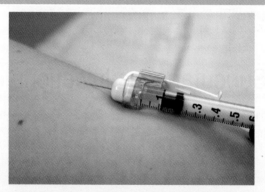

Inserting the needle almost level with the skin. (From Taylor, C., Lillis, C., LeMone, P., and Lynn, P. [2008]. *Fundamentals of nursing: The art and science of nursing care.* [6th ed.] Philadelphia: Lippincott Williams & Wilkins, p. 834.)

Gauge		Needle Length (in.)		Solution (mL)	
Range	*Average*	*Range*	*Average*	*Range*	*Average*
27–25	26	$\frac{3}{8}$ to $\frac{5}{8}$	$\frac{1}{2}$	0.1–0.5	<0.5

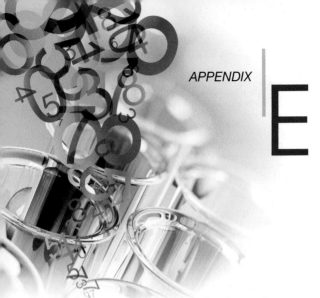

Subcutaneous Injections

The subcutaneous route is used for insulin and heparin.

The Subcutaneous Route

Use
- An insulin syringe
- A prefilled disposable syringe with appropriate needle length

Inject
Under the skin into the adipose tissue below the dermis

*Angle**
45–90 degrees

45°   90°

The Subcutaneous Route (continued)

Sites
Outer aspect of the upper arm (slow absorption), abdomen (rapid absorption), anterior part of thigh (very slow absorption), and upper dorsogluteal (slowest absorption).

*A 45-degree angle of insertion is used with a 5/8" needle for subcutaneous medications *except insulin and heparin*—for example, codeine sulfate and oxy-morphone hydrochloride. A 90-degree angle of insertion is used with a 3/8" to 1/2" needle for *insulin and heparin*.

Administering a Subcutaneous Injection

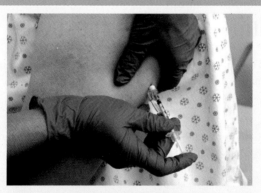

Bunching tissue around injection site. (From Taylor, C., Lillis, C., LeMone, P., and Lynn, P. [2008]. *Fundamentals of nursing: The art and science of nursing care* [6th ed.]. Philadelphia: Lippincott Williams & Wilkins, p. 837.)

Gauge		Needle Length (in.)		Solution (mL)	
Range	*Average*	*Range*	*Average*	*Range*	*Average*
28–23	26	$\frac{3}{8}$ to $\frac{5}{8}$	$\frac{3}{8}$ to $\frac{7}{8}$	0.2–2.0	<0.1

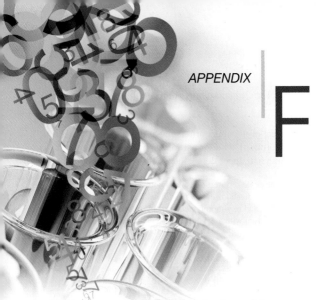

Intramuscular Injections

The *intramuscular route* is preferred for medications that:

- Are ineffectively absorbed in the gastrointestinal tract
- Require a more rapid onset of action than subcutaneous medications and may have a longer effect
- Can be administered in volumes up to 3.0 mL

The Intramuscular Route

Use
A 3.0-mL syringe

Inject
Into the body of a striated muscle. Inject past the dermis and subcutaneous tissue. Always aspirate before injecting.

The Intramuscular Route (continued)

Angle
Always 90 degrees

↓ 90°

Sites
Ventrogluteal, vastus lateralis, deltoid, and dorsogluteal.
Depends on patient's age and the volume of medication.

Administering an Intramuscular Injection

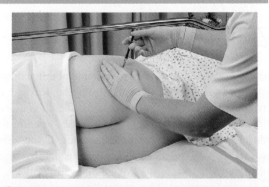

Spreading the skin at site and injecting medication at
90-degree angle. (From Taylor, C., Lillis, C., and LeMone, P.
[2001]. *Fundamentals of nursing: The art and science of
nursing care* [4th ed.]. Philadelphia: Lippincott Williams &
Wilkins, p. 607.)

Gauge		Needle Length (in.)		Solution (mL)	
Range	*Average*	*Range*	*Average*	*Range*	*Average*
25–20	22	1.0–2.0	1.5	0.5–5.0	1.0

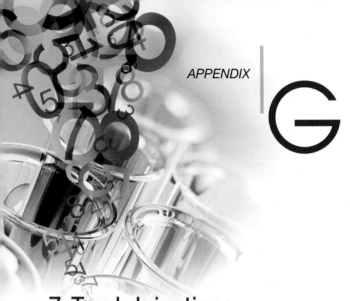

Z-Track Injections

The *Z-track* method is used for parenteral drug administration when tissue damage from the leakage of irritating medications is expected or when it is essential that all of the medication can be absorbed in the muscle and not in the subcutaneous tissue. The method is easy, popular, and recommended by some institutions as a safe way of administering all intramuscular injections. This method prevents "tracking" of the medication along the path of the needle during insertion and removal.

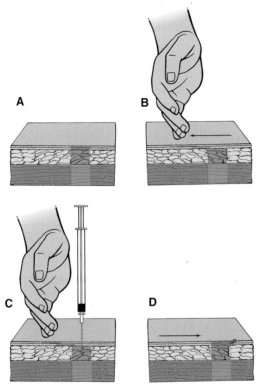

The Z-track or zigzag technique is recommended for intramuscular injections. **(A)** Normal skin and tissues. **(B)** Moving the skin to one side. **(C)** Needle is inserted at a 90-degree angle, and the nurse aspirates for blood. **(D)** Once the needle is withdrawn, displaced tissue is allowed to return to its normal position, preventing the solution from escaping from the muscle tissue. (From Taylor, C., Lillis, C., LeMone, P., and Lynn, P. [2008]. *Fundamentals of nursing: The art and science of nursing care* [6th ed.]. Philadelphia: Lippincott Williams & Wilkins, p. 840.)

The *Z*-Track Route

Use
A 3.0-mL syringe

Inject
Deep into the body of the gluteal muscle; the vastus lateralis can also be used.

Angle
Always 90 degrees

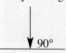

90°

Injection Technique
Displace or push tissue over muscle toward the center of the body by displacing the tissue with the last three fingers of the nondominant hand. Hold the tissues in this displaced position before, during, and for 5 to 15 seconds after the injection so the medication can begin to be absorbed. Use the IM injection technique as described in Appendix F.

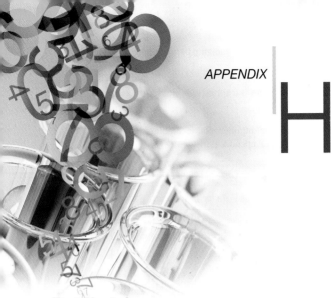

Pediatric Intramuscular Injections

The Intramuscular Route

Use

A needle about 1 inch in length. For infants a 5/8-inch needle may be used.

Inject

Into dense muscle mass in the deltoid and ventrogluteal muscles. Into the outer quadrant of the gluteal and vastus lateralis muscles.

Angle

Preferably 45 degrees. May use 90 degrees if the child's age and body mass warrant it.

The Intramuscular Route (continued)

Injection Technique
Similar to the intramuscular technique for adults as described in Appendix F.

Gauge		Needle Length (in.)		Solution (mL)	
Range	*Average*	*Range*	*Average*	*Range*	*Average*
22–20	22	0.5–1.5	1.0	0.5–2.5	0.5–1.0 (<3 yrs) 0.5–1.5 (4–6 yrs) 0.5–2.0 (7–14 yrs) 1.0–2.5 (>15 yrs)

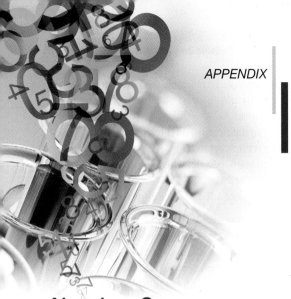

Nursing Concerns for Pediatric Drug Administration

When administering medications to children, you need to be aware of the following:

- Explain honestly what will be done; explain at the level of the child's understanding.
- Use supplemental materials to promote understanding (stuffed animals, dolls).
- Suggest that the child help as much as possible; encourage the child to pretend, and switch roles with the child.
- Reinforce positive behavior with praise and rewards if necessary.
- Make sure you have obtained an accurate height and weight measurement.

- Be sure that you have compared the safe dosage range with the dosage you plan to give; know toxic and lethal doses.
- Do not force medication on a frightened child, especially one who is crying.
- Always use two people when giving injections to small children.
- Disguise or dilute medications if necessary.

A nurse also needs to understand that the child's immature body system may respond differently to drugs, so there may be changes in an agent's absorption, distribution, biotransformation, and elimination. (See Appendix H for information about pediatric intramuscular injections.)

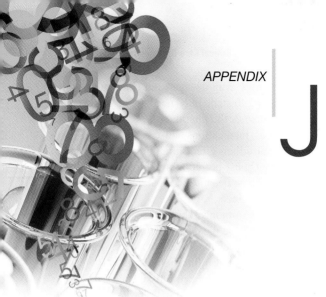

Nursing Considerations for Critical Care Drug Administration

A patient who is critically ill may experience rapid hemodynamic changes. The nurse must possess knowledge of the medications administered and the effect of these medications on vital signs. Therefore, the nurse needs to be aware of the following considerations when administering medications to a patient who is critically ill:

- Blood pressure, pulse, and heart rhythms must be monitored frequently to titrate medications based on prescribed parameters.
- Drugs may be given to increase blood pressure (vasopressors) or to decrease blood pressure (vasodilators).

- Calculation of drug dosages and flow rates, which can be complicated, may need to be checked by another nurse or the pharmacist.
- Intravenous medications must be monitored carefully because their effects are immediate.
- The patient must be monitored closely for adverse drug reactions because critical care medications have potent effects.
- Drugs are commonly started at a low dose and titrated to achieve the desired effect.
- Intravenous insertion sites must be monitored closely for signs of infiltration. Some vasopressors, such as dopamine, can cause tissue necrosis.
- Critical care patients commonly have multiple drug infusions running at the same time. The nurse must check drug compatibilities before administering two medications together in the same intravenous site.

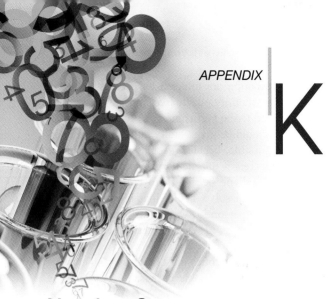

Nursing Concerns for Geriatric Drug Administration

As with pediatric medications, special consideration is given when administering drugs to anyone who is older than 65 years of age. This is because physiologic changes caused by aging change the way the body reacts to certain drugs. For example, a tranquilizer may increase restlessness and agitation in an elderly person.

You should be aware of the following general considerations before administering a drug to any elderly individual.

- Small, frail elderly individuals will probably require less than the normal adult dosages. Drug absorption and distribution are affected by decreased gastro-intestinal motility, decreased muscle mass, and diminished tissue perfusion.

- A drug should be given orally rather than parenterally, if possible, because decreased activity in the elderly decreases muscle tissue absorption.
- Often, it will be necessary to crush pills, empty capsules, or dissolve medications in liquid in order to assist the person to swallow without discomfort. Tell the patient *not to crush* enteric-coated or time-released drugs.
- Sedatives and narcotics must be given with extreme caution to elderly people because they may easily become oversedated.
- Because the elderly are often on many different medications, you should check for drug interactions that may cause hazardous effects (e.g., giving a sedative shortly after a tranquilizer).
- The cumulative side effects of the drugs being administered must be monitored. A drug's excretion may be altered if the patient has reduced renal blood flow and reduced kidney function.
- A schedule for rotation of injection sites should be followed carefully because the elderly have decreased muscle mass and increased vascular fragility.
- Any written directions for medication administration should be clear and in large print because of possible impaired vision.
- The problem of impaired hearing should be kept in mind when giving directions or asking questions. You may have to speak very loudly or repeat the same information several times.

Writing the directions is recommended for some patients.

- Reinforce any important information by asking the patient to repeat it for you. This also helps you to ascertain whether the information was understood. Memory loss and confusion are common in the elderly because of cerebral arteriosclerosis.

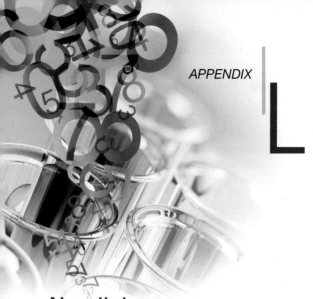

Needleless Intravenous System

Shown on the next page are a syringe being prepared to be injected into a needleless port and a piggyback setup connected to a needleless port. (Photo by Rick Brady.) (From Taylor, C., Lillis, C., LeMone, P., and Lynn, P. [2008]. *Fundamentals of nursing: The art and science of nursing care* [6th ed.]. Philadelphia: Lippincott Williams & Wilkins, pp. 792 and 851.)

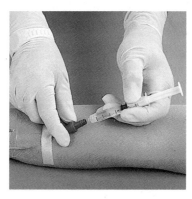

Syringe prepared to be injected into a needleless port.
(From Taylor, C., Lillis, C., LeMone, P., and Lynn, P. [2008].
Fundamentals of nursing: The art and science of nursing care
[6th ed.]. Philadelphia: Lippincott Williams & Wilkins, p. 792.)

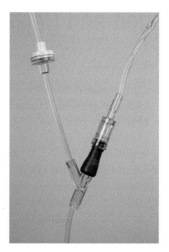

Piggyback setup connected to a needleless port. (From
Taylor, C., Lillis, C., LeMone, P., and Lynn, P. [2008].
Fundamentals of nursing: The art and science of nursing care
[6th ed.]. Philadelphia: Lippincott Williams & Wilkins, p. 851.)

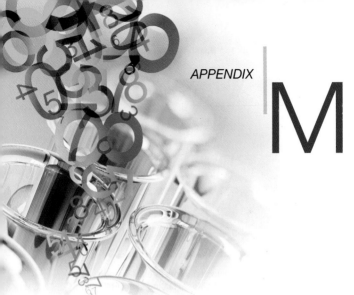

Temperature Conversions: Fahrenheit and Celsius Scales

Electronic digital thermometers that convert between temperature scales are popular. However, it is still necessary for health care practitioners to understand the differences between the scales and to be able to apply the conversion formulas.

The differences between the scales, as shown in the following table, are based on the differences between the boiling and freezing points. This difference, 180 (F) and 100 (C), forms the basis for the conversion formulas.

Scale	Abbreviation	Boiling Point	Freezing Point
Fahrenheit	F	212	32
Centigrade	C	100	0

RULE

To change from Fahrenheit to Celsius, perform the following steps:

- Subtract 32 degrees from the Fahrenheit reading.
- Divide by 9/5 (1.8) or, for convenience, multiply by 5/9.
- $C = (F - 32) \times \dfrac{5}{9}$

EXAMPLE: Convert 100°F to Celsius.

$$\begin{array}{r} 100 \\ -32 \\ \hline 68 \end{array} \qquad \frac{68}{1} \times \frac{5}{9} = \frac{340}{9}$$

$$= 340 \div 9 = 37.7°C$$

ANSWER: 37.7° Celsius

RULE

To change from Celsius to Fahrenheit, perform the following steps:

- Multiply the Celsius reading by 9/5 or 1.8.
- Add 32.
- $F = (9/5 \times C \text{ or } C \times 1.8) + 32$

EXAMPLE: Convert 40°C to Fahrenheit.

$$\cancel{40}^{8} \times \frac{9}{\cancel{5}_{1}} = 72$$

or

$$40 \times 1.8 = 72$$

$$\begin{array}{r} 72 \\ +32 \\ \hline 104° \end{array}$$

ANSWER: 104° Fahrenheit

You may find the following temperature conversion scale useful for quick reference.

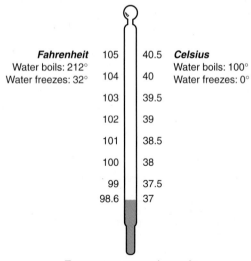

Fahrenheit			*Celsius*
Water boils: 212°	105	40.5	Water boils: 100°
Water freezes: 32°	104	40	Water freezes: 0°
	103	39.5	
	102	39	
	101	38.5	
	100	38	
	99	37.5	
	98.6	37	

Temperature conversion scale

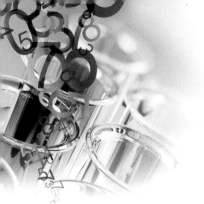

Index

Page numbers followed by app indicate appendices; page numbers followed by f indicate figures; and t following a page number indicates tabular material.